Secrets of the Pulse

Secrets of the Pulse

The Ancient Art of
Ayurvedic Pulse Diagnosis
Second Edition

by

Dr. Vasant Dattatray Lad

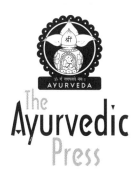

Albuquerque, New Mexico

The Ayurvedic Press
Albuquerque, New Mexico

Although the information contained in this book is based on Ayurvedic principles practiced for thousands of years, it should not be taken or construed as standard medical diagnosis or treatment. For any medical condition, always consult with a qualified physician.

Sanskrit passages translated by Vasant Lad.
All illustrations and drawings by Vasant Lad.
Cover design by Michael Quanci.
Layout by Laura Humphreys.
Edited by Margaret Smith Peet. Revision editors Glen Crowther and Barbara Cook.

Library of Congress Cataloging-in-Publication Data

Lad, Vasant, 1943-
    Secrets of the pulse : the ancient art of ayurvedic pulse diagnosis /
  by Vasant Dattatray Lad. -- 2nd ed.
      p. cm.
    Summary: "A resource on learning ayurvedic pulse diagnosis, including the seven levels of the pulse and its interpretations of disease and health. Offers detailed techniques for learning to evaluate the radial pulse while explaining the ayurvedic understanding of the body's systems, its disorders and how to correct them" --Provided by publisher.
    Includes bibliographical references.
    ISBN-13: 978-1-883725-13-6 (pbk. : alk. paper)
    ISBN-10: 1-883725-13-5 (pbk. : alk. paper)
    1. Pulse. 2. Physical diagnosis. 3. Medicine, Ayurvedic.   I. Title.
RC74.L33 2006
616.07'54--dc22
                                        2005036262

Published by **The Ayurvedic Press** • 11311 Menaul Blvd NE • Albuquerque, NM 87112-0008
For more information on Ayurveda, contact:
The Ayurvedic Institute
11311 Menaul Blvd. NE
Albuquerque, NM 87112
(505)291-9698 • Fax 505.294.7572 • www.ayurveda.com

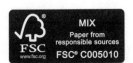

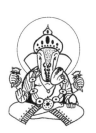

॥ श्रीः ॥

This book is dedicated with all my
heart to my loving wife, Ushā, who
has inspired and supported me in all
walks of my life.

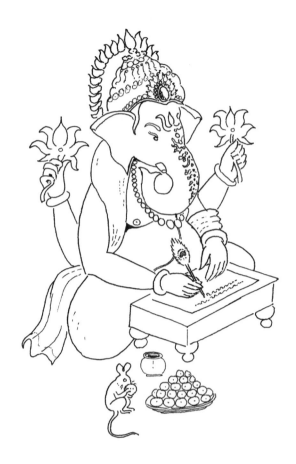

Lord Ganesha
ॐ गँ गणपतये नमः ।

Salutation to Lord Ganesha who is the seed of wisdom and light.

(translation of sūtra)

Lord Ganesha first wrote the story of human life in the form of the Mahabharata, dictated to Him by Maharshi Vyāsa, which later became the true history of mankind, revealing various potentials and characteristics of human beings. With His love and blessings one may learn the hidden secrets of the pulse as written in this book.

Ganesha is the son of Shiva and Parvati. He is the first Lord to be worshipped at the beginning of any auspicious work. He removes obstacles and brings success, fulfillment and great joy to the life of every human being.

Table of Contents

List of Illustrations

List of Tables

The Use of Sanskrit

Knowledge of Āyurveda originates in the Sanskrit language. Sanskrit is a precise phonetic language that uses a set of written symbols not familiar to most Westerners. The phonetic representation of Sanskrit words using the English alphabet is called transliteration. We can transliterate Sanskrit to English characters, but not every sound translates directly. There are quite a few sounds that do not exist in the English language, requiring special characters to represent them accurately.

One example is वात, which translates to vāta. The first 'a' in vāta is a 'long a', as in "father"; it is held for two beats. The second 'a' is a 'short a', as in "what." Another example is a sound somewhere between an 'i', a 'u' and an 'r' that occurs in the word प्रकृतिं. This word is transliterated as prakṛti. The 'ṛ' is pronounced as the 'ri' in the English spelling of the word Krishna. To make things even more complicated, among those who use Sanskrit the 'ṛ' is pronounced in northern India as the 'i' in "it" and in southern India as the 'u' sound in "root." Because of the regional variations in pronunciation, in this book both ru and ri are found in place of the technically correct 'ṛ'.

Another consideration is that the trailing 'a' in Sanskrit words is sometimes omitted because of the influence of the Hindi language. It is included in many of the words in this book. The trailing 'a' is also subject to grammatical changes depending on the letters that follow it and, for simplicity's sake, we generally ignore these rules. For example, the word *meda* (fat) can be transliterated as *medo, medas,* and meda depending on the word following it. Ordinarily, we use the most common form, meda, so that you, the reader, will have to learn only the one word. Of course, it would be wonderful if all our readers began the study of Sanskrit, inspired by the knowledge available in these ancient texts, but it is not our purpose here to teach that language.

In *Secrets of the Pulse* we have chosen to use transliteration characters only for long vowels, denoted by an overscore or macron character, and for the 'nya' sound denoted by 'ñ'. The pronunciations of the vowels are:

a as in about; **ā** as in father
i as in ink; **ī** as in fee
u as in put; **ū** as in food
e as in pay; **ai** as in I
o as in corn; **au** as in loud

This new edition contains revisions and expanded descriptions that developed in response to the questions and feedback of many students and teachers who use this book in classroom and clinical settings in Ayurveda schools and clinics around the world. We hope these changes enhance the reader's integration of the information.

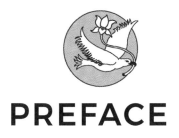

PREFACE

Since 1982, I have been traveling extensively giving lectures on various aspects of Ayurveda. Because of the interest in Ayurveda in the hearts of both practitioners and laymen and because of the demand, I have also been teaching seminars on pulse diagnosis across the United States, England and at the Ayurvedic Institute in Albuquerque, New Mexico.

In any system of medicine, pulse assessment is a matter of technical skill, subjective experience and intuition. Accuracy also depends upon the individual's persistent practice and quality of sensitive awareness. My early education in pulse reading was influenced by several teachers, gurus and yogis in India. Even though simplified descriptions of various conditions of the pulse are found in the standard Ayurvedic texts, the methods of examination are not given in detail. However, it is possible to learn these subjective methods of pulse examination that reveal the characteristics of the individual's prakruti, vikruti and various doshic disorders and to verify their accuracy objectively.

During my travels, many students encouraged me to write a book on pulse diagnosis based upon Ayurvedic principles. The purpose of this book is to teach simplified techniques to students and to provide deep comprehensive information as well. Throughout my earlier Ayurvedic education, I also studied modern allopathic medicine and this knowledge has broadened my interpretation of pulse reading. It is quite interesting to note that Charaka and Sushruta, well known Ayurvedic physician and surgeon, respectively, say:

तस्माच्छास्त्रेऽर्थे विज्ञाने प्रवृत्तौ कर्म दर्शने ।

भिषक् चतुष्ट्ये युक्तः प्राणाभिसर उच्यते ॥ १८ ॥

च. सू. ९

Therefore, the physician who possesses the four-fold accomplishment consisting of theoretical knowledge, clear interpretation, right application and practical experience is to be regarded as the reclaimer of life.

Ca. Sū. 9:18

एकं शास्त्रमधीयानो न विद्याच्छास्त्र निश्चयम् ।

तस्माद् बहुश्रुतः शास्त्रं विजानीयाच्चिकित्सकः ॥ ७ ॥

सु.सू. ४

*By knowing one science alone, one cannot arrive at an accurate
scientific assessment. Therefore, a physician should study other
sciences in order to arrive at correct diagnosis.*

Su. Sū. 4:7

प्रयोगज्ञानविज्ञानसिद्धिसिद्धाः सुखप्रदाः ।

जीविताभिसराये स्युर्वैद्यत्वं तेष्ववस्थितमिति ॥ ५३ ॥

च. सू. ११

*Those who are accomplished in application, theory, knowledge of
allied sciences and success of treatment are the true healers. In
them is the glory of the physician fully manifest.*

Ca. Sū. 11:53

These quotes from the Vedic texts show that Ayurveda is an all-inclusive science of life and is open to all avenues of healing.

All of what I am sharing with you in this book may not be found in the standard Ayurvedic texts. However, all that I have included here is based upon Ayurvedic principles. I received this knowledge from my mentors in the Ayurvedic tradition and it has since unfolded in my heart through clinical observation and practice over the last 35 years.

This book will give guidelines to think about various ways of feeling, reading and gathering information through the pulse. It is quite difficult to put subjective experience into words. This is my sincere attempt to express these simple ways of feeling the pulse. I hope, dear readers, that you will love this humble effort.

Love and light,

Dr. Vasant Lad
Albuquerque, New Mexico
May 1996

Acknowledgments

The author would like to acknowledge those whose dedication and insight brought the knowledge of Ayurveda to the world, especially his teachers who lovingly showed the way and shared their knowledge and experience, and all the friends and staff at the Ayurvedic Institute without whose contributions this book would not exist. Finally, and with deep gratitude, the author would like to acknowledge the work of Margaret Smith Peet who tirelessly transcribed and edited the vast amount of material for this book.

NĀDI VIJÑĀNAM
The Art of Reading the Pulse

प्रकृतिं पश्यति पुरुषः प्रेक्षकवदवस्थितः स्वस्थः ।६५।
सां.का.

Remaining stable in one's own state of being,
Purusha, the soul, witnesses Prakruti, the creation.
Sān. Kâ. 65

The entire Vedic tradition is composed of highly spiritual wisdom and pure knowledge revealed through the hearts of enlightened *rishis* (sages). It is not a creation made by the mind of man, but rather unfolded in the hearts of meditative beings. The ancient Vedic wisdom came from the caves and mountains of India, where the rishis had ashrams and disciples. Students came to study in the *guru's* home. The rishis imparted knowledge as they experienced it in a deep state of meditation. These early teachings were an oral tradition and, because there were no books, the students stored the knowledge in their brains and it became a part of them.

The knowledge of *Āyurveda* has been passed down to us in *sūtras*, or small phrases, and the wisdom they contain is there to be unlocked by the inquiring mind. Much of the information in this book is based upon the truths contained in these ancient sūtras, which were written in the form of poetry during Vedic times more than 5,000 years ago. The Sanskrit word sūtra literally means 'to suture with a thread'. The words of a sūtra convey veiled subconscious meaning to consciousness. However, the discovery of these secret meanings needs the guidance of a teacher. The phrase of the sūtra is analogous to a thread passing through the eye of a needle. The eye of the needle is small, but the trail of the thread leads to great hidden wisdom waiting for interpretation.

"Āyur-Veda," translated as "The Science of Life," is an Upa-Veda, or secondary Veda, to the four main Vedas—Samaveda, Yajurveda, Atharvaveda and Rigveda—that are among the oldest bodies of knowledge in human culture. The knowledge contained in Āyurveda deals with the nature, scope and purpose of life. It embraces metaphysical and physical, health and disease, happiness and sorrow, pain and pleasure. It defines life as the expression of Cosmic Consciousness, as exemplified by the entire sphere of creation. Stated simply, the purpose of life is to know or realize the Creator (Cosmic Consciousness) and to express this divinity in one's daily life.

Āyurveda incorporates the six systems of Indian philosophy—Nyāya, Vaisheshika, Sānkhya, Yoga, Mīmāmsā and Vedanta. Later, Āyurveda also included Buddhism. Sānkhya philosophy, the system most basic to Āyurveda, outlines a model of creation and evolution. The sages discovered truth through intensive meditation. Āyurveda is a science of daily living that evolved from the rishis' practical, philosophical and spiritual illumination, which was rooted in their understanding of creation. They perceived how cosmic energy manifests in all living and non-living things. They also realized that the source of all existence is Universal Consciousness, which manifests as male and female energy—*Purusha* and *Prakruti*.

The rishi Kapila, the founder of Sānkhya philosophy, discerned 24 principles or elements in the manifestation of the universe. Purusha is said to be male and Prakruti is female. Purusha is formless, colorless, beyond attributes and takes no active part in creation. It is choiceless, passive awareness. Prakruti yields form, color and attributes in the field of action. It is awareness with choice, Divine Will, the One who desires to become many. The universe is a child born out of the womb of Prakruti, the Divine Mother. Prakruti creates all forms in the universe, while Purusha is the witness to this creation.

The three *gunas* of *sattva* (pure essence), *rajas* (movement) and *tamas* (inertia) are the universal qualities within all existence and are contained in Prakruti. When their equilibrium is disturbed, there is an interaction of the gunas which thus engenders the evolution of the universe. Rajas is the active vital life force in the body that moves both the organic and inorganic universal aspects to sattva and tamas, respectively. So sattva and tamas are inactive, potential energies that require the active, kinetic force of rajas. Sattva is creative potential (Brahma); rajas is kinetic protective force (Vishnu); and tamas is resistance to change or potential destructive force (Mahesvara). Creation (Brahma), Protection (Vishnu) and Change or Destruction (Mahesvara) are the three manifestations of the first cosmic soundless sound, *aum*, which are constantly operating in the universe. The illustration at right shows the manifestation of creation according to Sānkhya.

Sānkhya ~ The Flow of Consciousness and the Pulse

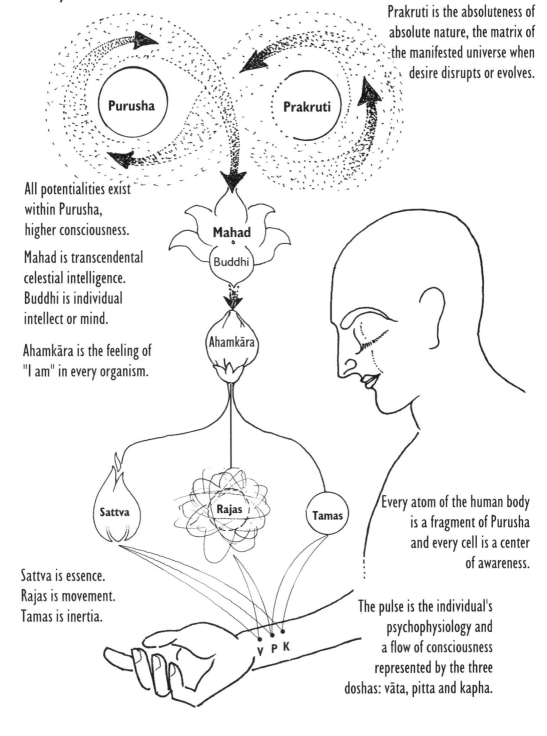

Prakruti is the absoluteness of absolute nature, the matrix of the manifested universe when desire disrupts or evolves.

Purusha

Prakruti

All potentialities exist within Purusha, higher consciousness.

Mahad is transcendental celestial intelligence. Buddhi is individual intellect or mind.

Ahamkāra is the feeling of "I am" in every organism.

Mahad
Buddhi

Ahamkāra

Sattva

Rajas

Tamas

Sattva is essence.
Rajas is movement.
Tamas is inertia.

Every atom of the human body is a fragment of Purusha and every cell is a center of awareness.

The pulse is the individual's psychophysiology and a flow of consciousness represented by the three doshas: vāta, pitta and kapha.

V P K

The first expression of Prakruti is *Mahad*, intelligence. From Mahad the ego (*Ahamkāra*) is formed, which is the sense of "I am." Ahamkāra then manifests into the five senses, five motor organs and the mind (*manas*) with the help of sattva and rajas, thus creating the organic universe. Ahamkāra further manifests into the five subtle tanmātrās and then into the five basic elements (Space, Air, Fire, Water and Earth) with the help of rajas and tamas, to create the inorganic universe.

सेन्द्रियं चेतनं द्रव्यं निरिन्द्रियमचेतनम् ॥ ४८ ॥
च. सू. १-

Substances endowed with sensory organization are organic (or sentient) and others, which are not endowed, are inorganic (or non-sentient).

Ca. Sū. 1:48

Āyurveda is the art of daily living in harmony with the laws of nature. Its aims and objectives are to maintain the perfect health of a healthy person through prevention of disease and to cure the disease process in an unhealthy person, through the use of proper diet, lifestyle, *panchakarma* cleansing and rejuvenation. For this purpose, we need a basic understanding of pulse diagnosis. The pulse technique is called *nādi vijñānam*. *Nādi* means pulse and *vijñānam* means understanding or specialized knowledge.

Āyurveda is a practical, clinical, medical science. Part of its unique methodology involves eight clinical examinations: pulse, urine, feces, eyes, tongue, speech, skin and form. The most important of these is the pulse, the foremost clinical art that Āyurveda has used through the ages. An experienced Āyurvedic physician will assess *prakruti*, *vikruti*, *doshic* disorders, other subtle observations and even prognosis of disease through the pulse. Āyurvedic pulse assessment opens up the doors of perception to explore the hidden secrets of life.

Pulse is a subtle manifestation of universal consciousness that pulsates through a person's constitution. As we know, the pulsation of blood through the body carries nutrients to the cellular level. There is a continuous flow of communication between cells, and this flow of communication is intelligence. The pulse can reveal cellular intelligence through a person's constitution.

The Sanskrit literature contains a number of words that can be translated as pulse. The most commonly used word is nādi, which means a river of life expressed through the pulse. The second synonym for pulse is *snāyu*, literally translated as subcutaneous tissue or fascia. As we know, the pulse lies within the subcutaneous tissue, so it is sometimes called snāyu. The third word is *tantu*, which means the string of a musical instrument, through which one can listen to the music of feelings and emotions.

Another synonym is *hamsa vahini*, or *hamsī*. In the breath, there is a sound called "*so-hum*" or "*ham-sa*." "*So*" goes with the inhalation and "*hum*" with exhalation.[1] *Hamsa* is actually a male swan and hamsī is a female swan. The sound vibrations of the breath move through the nādis, so the pulse is called hamsī. When "ham-sa, ham-sa, ham-sa" is repeated, it eventually becomes "so-hum, so-hum, so-hum." "So" is Shiva, while "hum" is *Shakti* and "sohum" represents the union of Shiva and Shakti. The entire universe is an expression of the union of Shiva and Shakti. These ancient deities of India, representing male and female energy, are really one; likewise, "so-hum" and "ham-sa" are the same. It is natural to inhale "so" and exhale "hum." "So" is higher consciousness, which goes inward. "Hum" is the ego, which goes out.

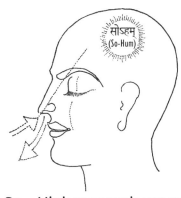

So = Higher consciousness
Hum = Individual Self

This divine mantra is constantly occurring through the breath of every living being. Each time we breathe in, the sound "so" goes in, and the sound "hum" goes out each time we exhale. So-hum means "I am that," beyond limitation of mind and body. "I am one with the Absolute."

Another synonym for the pulse is *dhamanī*. Dhamanī means artery, the pulsating blood vessel that carries blood away from the heart. During cardiac activity, the heart produces the sound "dhum-dhum" and, through each dhamanī, prāna is supplied to all the *dhātus* (tissues). *Dhāranī* means to hold or support. The pulse moves through all organs, so it is also called dhāranī, meaning "that which holds all the organs together," or "that which holds life." Pulse is also called *dhārā*, which means the continuous flow of consciousness; *sarita*, a river of daily life; and *jīva*, the expression of individual life.

There are other usages of the word nādi. *Vishva* means universe, so the flow of universal energy is called *vishva nādi*, which is connected to individual life through *prāna* and the breath in particular. Sit quietly and bring total attention to the breath. Try to detect which nostril has the most air passing through it. Then note the subtle sensation where the air is brushing against the inner nostril. The breath of the right nostril is male solar energy; the left nostril breath is lunar energy, which is female. Approximately every 90 minutes, the breath pattern changes, alternating between breathing through the right nostril and the left.

When the exhalation and inhalation of air mainly brush the inner sides of the nostrils, the Earth element is activated, creating a feeling of groundedness and stability. On the other hand, when the air brushes the sides of the nostrils near the cheeks, the Water element is working and one will feel emotional, compassionate and loving. When the

---

1.   Technically, the proper spelling is "so-ham." To avoid students mis-pronouncing this, Dr. Lad always spells it "so-hum." In deference to this custom, we continue to spell it "so-hum."

breath touches more towards the tip of the nostrils, the Fire element is activated and one is prone to feel fiery, judgmental, critical, ambitious and competitive. The Air element is active when the breath touches the outer sides of the nostrils, causing a fluctuating, hyperactive and confused mind. When Space element is prominent, the breath is subtle, neither touching the right nor left sides of the nostrils, but coming from the central axis of the nose, creating tranquility and peace. These cosmic elements of Space, Air, Fire, Water and Earth are communicated to the individual life through the breath and vishva nādi.

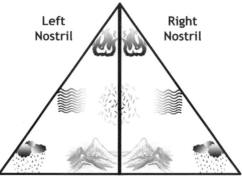

Left Nostril   **Right Nostril**

Table 1: Elements in the Breath

MANTRA	SYMBOL	ELEMENT	EMOTIONS
Hām		Space or Ether	Tranquility, peace, freedom, isolation, loneliness
Yam		Air	Hyperactivity, confusion, fear, anxiety, fluctuation of emotions
Rām		Fire	Competition, aggression, judgment, violence
Vam		Water	Love, compassion, attachment, greed
Lam		Earth	Groundedness, stability, depression, heaviness

Another nādi that appears in the *shāstras* is called *guru nādi*. Guru means master, teacher, or enlightened being. At the time of initiation, the guru "looks" into the initiate's third eye, making certain gestures called *mudrās*, and with the thumb gives *shaktipāta* (energy transmission), which awakens the guru nādi and intuition in that person. When the guru nādi starts pulsating, prakruti and vikruti become balanced. This balanced state of being opens the *sushumnā*, the central pathway in the spine, creating a state of transformation. Blessed are those whose guru nādi is awakened. It is a spiritual

Guru nādi

phenomenon that has to be received from a guru. When the guru nādi is working, awakening of *kundalinī shakti* takes place. Guru nādi is the basis of universal polarity, the balancing of opposite principles within an individual.

When the guru nādi is awakened, one can feel one's own pulse and through that pulse, while "looking" into the third eye of another person, can feel what is happening with that other person. "Look" directly into the third eye of the person whose pulse you are taking. Make your mind completely empty and, in that emptiness, begin to welcome and visualize whatever comes. Feel what is happening to the subject as you bring awareness to the tips of the fingers. This is a state of effortless awareness. The art of emptiness is the art of awareness and the guru nādi takes expression through this timeless state. We have to see things as a whole and not give emphasis to one fragment. Truth is whole and reality is localized. See as a whole and then go to the root cause. This approach sounds rather exotic, however Āyurveda gives us logic and then helps us to go beyond that logic.

The synonyms discussed above describe different aspects of the pulse. There are two more Sanskrit words associated with the pulse found in the literature: *prānāchārya* and *dhanvantari*, meaning, respectively, one who uses prāna and higher states of consciousness for healing. For thousands of years, Vedic literature has used nādi as a common word for pulse and it is the most popular term for pulse in Āyurveda. Therefore, in this text, the pulse is referred to as nādi and the art or science of pulse reading is called nādi vijñānam.

NĀDI PREDICTION

Āyurveda uses *darshana*, *sparshana* and *prashna* as its main clinical barometers and nādi vijñānam relates to sparshana. Darshana means pure observation and it indicates optical perception or inspection, while prashna is questioning. Sparshana is the tactile experience of touch.

The body, mind and spirit exist together in daily life as one unit, just as all things in the universe exist together in harmony. In reality, we are consciousness, pure awareness, and the body is an expression of that consciousness. One way of creating that quality of pure awareness is to simultaneously pay attention to the outer object and the inner movement of sensation. Then the *tanmātrās* are revealed. There

वातं पित्तं कफं द्वन्द्वं त्रितयं सान्निपातिकम् ।
साध्यासाध्यविवेकं च सर्वं नाडी प्रकाशयेत्
॥ ४८ ॥
यो. र. १

Pulse denotes vāta-pitta-kapha, their dual and triple disorders, as well as expresses prognosis of diseases.
Yoga Ratnakar, 1:48

are five elements—Ether, Air, Fire, Water, Earth—and they each have a respective tanmātrā. Sound is the subtle tanmātrā of Space, touch is the tanmātrā of Air, vision or sight of Fire, taste of Water, and odor or smell is the tanmātrā of Earth. Hence the grosser five elements are merged into five subtle tanmātrās. An outer object stimulates the senses, through which the mind touches the outer object by way of the tanmātrās. By that bridge, we experience perception.

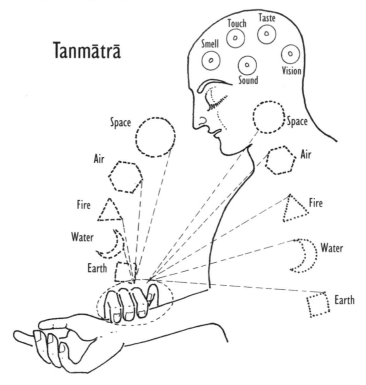

Tanmātrā

Our mind consists of five tanmātric substances. External sound stimulates the inner *shabda tanmātrā* of the mind, which meets the outer sound. There is also touch, vision, taste and smell in the mind. We are constantly touching the outer environment through the sensations of touch. Through the skin, touch stimulates the inner mental faculty of *sparsha*. The examination of pulse is related to *sparsha tanmātrā*, which is associated with the sense of touch. In a way, a tanmātrā is a vehicle. By the tanmātrās, our consciousness goes out and touches the objects of our perception. So the five tanmātrās of sound, touch, sight, taste and smell are used by Āyurvedic physicians (*vaidyas*) to diagnose any problem. These five tanmātrās are our doors of perception, our innermost instruments of experience.

अर्थे दश महामूलाः समासक्ता महाफलाः ।
महच्चार्थिश्च हृदयं पयायैरुच्यते बुधैः ॥ ३ ॥
च. सू. ३०

There are ten vessels of great biological importance attached to the heart. Mahad, artha and hridaya are the synonyms.

Ca. Sū. 30:3

The radial pulse, which is the pulse of the radial artery in the forearm, is usually chosen as the site to read the pulse. This is because it is convenient and more readily available than other pulse sites. The radial pulse reveals the characteristics of doshic imbalance, the nature of any diseases and their expected prognosis.

The pulsation of the radial artery corresponds to the heart beat and the heart is the center of the five tanmātrās. When I say the word "heart," it means not just the physical heart, but also a center in our innermost being from which we perceive.

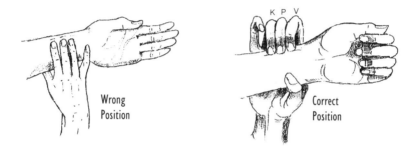

Wrong Position

Correct Position

PULSE TECHNIQUE

Always feel the pulse from the radial side of the arm and never from the ulnar side. When viewing the hand in the anatomical position of the body, the radial side is near the thumb and the ulnar side runs down from the little finger. On the radial side there is a bony protuberance called the radial tubercle. There are two schools of thought about finger placement when taking a person's pulse. The index finger can either be placed above or below the radial tubercle. However, if the finger is placed above the radial tubercle, a gap is created between the distal and middle fingers, so some authorities say to avoid the radial tubercle. The index finger is never placed on the radial tubercle, because this position will give an incorrect reading. I prefer keeping all three fingers together and proximal to the radial tubercle, which means closer to the heart. Do not bunch the fingers tightly, but separate them slightly, so that the throbbing under each finger can be felt distinctly.

Gap created by index finger being placed above the radial tubercle.

If the radial pulse is difficult to detect, first check the position of the hand (see illustration above) to be sure the finger placement is correct and in contact with the radial artery. In some people, this pulse may be perceptible only on one arm. In *kapha* individuals, obese people, and those with generalized swelling, the nādi is buried under adipose tissue. When reading the radial pulse, turn the neck of the subject to the side and look at the carotid artery and external jugular vein, to see if the jugular is pulsating or the carotid is dancing. A dancing carotid and nodding of the head can be a sign of an

षडङ्गमङ्गं विज्ञानमिन्द्रियाण्यर्थपञ्चकम् ।
आत्मा च सगुणश्चेतश्चिन्त्यं च हृदि संश्रितम् ॥ ४ ॥
च. सू. ३०

*The body with its six limbs,
understanding, the senses, five sense
objects, consciousness, mind and its
attributes are all dependent on the heart.*

Ca. Sū. 30:4

anomaly related to the heart, such as aortic regurgitation. Also touch the carotid, temporal and femoral pulses. Using darshana and sparshana together in this way, one can see and feel various changes taking place.

In the pulse at the temple, one finds out the condition of *prana vāta*, *sādhaka pitta* and *tarpaka kapha*, and their connection to *sahasrāra*. *Udāna vāyu*, *prāna vāyu*, *avalambaka kapha* and *rañjaka pitta* can be felt through the carotid. The brachial artery reveals the condition of *samāna vāyu*, *kledaka kapha* and *pāchaka pitta*. The femoral artery shows the pulsation of *apāna vāyu*, pāchaka pitta and *shleshaka kapha*, and the condition of the reproductive organs. Detailed discussion of these pulses can be found in Chapter Nine.

First, learn to monitor the pulse on one side at a time, using the right arm of a man and the left for a woman. However, after some practice, one should learn to feel the radial pulse on both sides of the subject simultaneously. When the subject is breathing better through the right nostril, then his or her right pulse is more prominent than the left, and vice versa. It depends on where the prāna energy is moving. There may also be a physiological cause for any imbalance. For example, an enlarged lymph node under the armpit may press the artery, creating a feeble pulse on that side.

As a whole, when a person has more male energy, the right pulse will be more prominent. If female energy is more strongly activated, the left pulse will be more prominent. The same thing is true in pregnancy. When the right pulse is more prominent, the conceived fetus is male. If the left is more prominent, the conceived fetus is female. This pulse indicates the polarity of male and female energy. When the polarity changes, the amplitude of the pulse changes. This change in the pulse depends upon the breathing pattern. If the person has more prominence in right cycle breathing, the right hand pulse will be stronger than the left, and vice versa. Feeling the pulse also reflects the polarity between the observer and the observed.

The left brain is masculine, governing all activity of the right side of the body. The right brain is feminine, which governs all activity on the left side. Prāna shifts from the right hemisphere to the left hemisphere. When the right brain is active, there is more female energy and the person is more compassionate, intuitive and loving. When a poet writes a poem, he uses the right part of the brain and the left pulse will be prominent. On the other hand, the left brain is masculine, male energy, which is mathematical, calculating, judgmental, critical and scientific. When a scientist is working in the laboratory and observing through a microscope, the left brain is active. The analytical left brain leads to ambition and competitiveness and when the left brain is active, the right pulse becomes prominent.

In deep meditation the primordial brain is activated. When in deep meditation, one enters into a neutral state that is neither male nor female. At that moment, the right and left nostrils breathe equally. There is a bridge between the right and left brain in the third ventricle called *chidākāsha*. Within the brain space, one can see a fountain of light moving along the spine. This river of light moves upward and passes through the marble of light, merging into the third ventricle, where one can see the blue pearl. This is not a romantic, poetic concept. It is the ultimate reality within you, the purpose of human birth and life, which is to become enlightened.

The fourth ventricle is shaped like a diamond. At the bottom is the central canal of the spinal cord and at the top is *rishi kesha*. *Kesha* means hair and rishi means 'seer of the mantra'. The land of the Vedas is within each person. Merely going to India, shaving one's head and putting on a loin cloth will never transform a person. One may look like a spiritual person but it is a superficial change. The real change is evident within the third ventricle of the brain. At the moment of enlightenment, both the right and left pulses become harmoniously identical, equal, gentle and balanced in both the superficial and deep pulses.

अग्रे वातवहा नाडी मध्ये वहति पित्तला ।
अन्ते श्लेष्मविकारेण नाडी ज्ञेया बुधैः सदा ॥५४॥
यो. र. १

Under the first, the index finger, vāta nāḍi occurs, while pitta appears beneath the middle finger and kapha ultimately shows below the ring finger. The wise person should always know these basic characteristics of pulse.

Yoga Ratnakar, 1:54

General Characteristics of Vāta, Pitta and Kapha Pulses

Ether[1], Air, Fire, Water and Earth, the five basic elements, manifest in the human body as three basic principles known as *doshas*. From the Ether and Air elements, the bodily air principle called *vāta* is manifested. The Fire and Water elements exist together as the fire principle called *pitta*. The Earth and Water elements exhibit as *kapha dosha*. These three doshas determine an individual's constitution and govern the functions of the body. When out of balance, they contribute to the disease process.

Before going into the actual study of the pulse, we will discuss the general characteristics of each doshic pulse. The rishis described the manner in which the pulse moved by comparing it to the movements of different animals. They called this movement *gati*. The mobility of the vāta pulse is called *sarpa gati* (cobra pulse), that of pitta is called *mandūka gati* (frog pulse), while the motion of kapha pulse is called *hamsa gati* (swan pulse).

---

1. The words "ether" and "space" are used interchangeably.

Vāta pulse is superficial, cold, light, thin, feeble and empty. With more pressure, it disappears. It moves fast and may become irregular. It is best felt under the index finger. With keen observation, one can feel a little leech or cobra moving under the finger. Try to have that insight when feeling the pulse. Vāta pulse is cold to the touch because of insufficient subcutaneous fat, which is why people with a vāta constitution lose heat and hate the cold.

Pitta pulse is full with a strong throb. It is hot and abrupt, with high amplitude, good volume and considerable force. It is best felt under the middle finger and it moves like a leaping frog. Pitta pulse is hot to the touch because pitta people have strong digestive fire and more heat.

Kapha pulse is deep, slow, watery, wavy and cool to the touch. It moves like a swimming swan. Kapha people retain heat in the body because of their thick layer of fat under the skin.

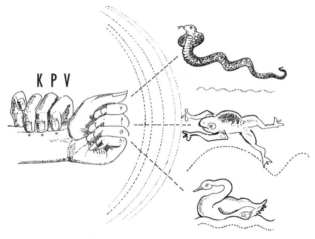

Table 2: Basic Qualities of the Pulse

	VĀTA PULSE	**PITTA PULSE**	**KAPHA PULSE**
Characteristics	Fast, feeble, cold, light, thin, disappears on pressure	Prominent, strong, high amplitude, hot, forceful, lifts up the palpating fingers	Deep, slow, broad, wavy, thick, cool or warm, regular
Location	Best felt under the index finger	Best felt under the middle finger	Best felt under the ring finger
Gati (Movement)	Moves like a cobra	Moves like a frog	Moves like a swimming swan

The temperature of the pulse denotes much more than just the feeling of warmth or cold felt on the skin. To the sensitive clinician, there is an intuitive feeling of temperature reflected through the pulse.

Vāta, pitta and kapha pulses are the three basic pulses considered in this text. We will also be using the terms proximal, middle and distal to refer to the positioning of each finger when taking the pulse. When correctly placed on the wrist, the ring finger, which is closest to the heart, is proximal. The index finger, which is away from the heart, is distal. In the middle position is the middle finger.

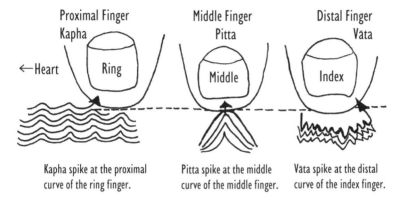

Proximal Finger	Middle Finger	Distal Finger
Kapha	Pitta	Vāta
←Heart Ring	Middle	Index

Kapha spike at the proximal curve of the ring finger.   Pitta spike at the middle curve of the middle finger.   Vāta spike at the distal curve of the index finger.

Thus, we have described finger placement and the general characteristics of the vāta, pitta and kapha pulses. An outline of the principle traits of each of these pulses is included in "Basic Qualities of the Pulse" on page 12.

Table 3: Seven Characteristics of the Pulse

	VĀTA	**PITTA**	**KAPHA**
Gati (Movement)	Sarpa (cobra)	Mandūka (frog)	Hamsa (swan)
Vega (Rate)	80-95	70-80	50-60
Tāla (Rhythm)	Irregular	Regular	Regular
Bala (Force)	Low +	High +++	Moderate ++
Ākruti (Tension and Volume)	Low	High	Moderate
Tapamāna (Temperature)	Cold	Hot	Warm to cool
Kāthinya (Consistency of Vessel Wall)	Rough, hard	Elastic, flexible	Soft, thickening

GATI (MOVEMENT)

The word gati means movement. In order to begin to understand the variety and complexity in pulse reading, we will look at some variations of the basic pulses or gatis.

This introduction will begin to expand our sensitivity and later we will go into the detection of specific disease conditions in more detail.

In addition to the three doshic gatis, there are other movements of the pulse that help to identify specific diseases. For example, in *jalauka gati* (leech pulse), the pulse touches the fingers of the clinician one after another in a rhythm like the movement of a leech (see illustration). This indicates that pitta has entered *rakta dhātu*, which then carries pitta deeper into

Jalauka Gati (Leech Pulse)

asthi dhātu (the joints), leading to gout and arthritis. Also under the heading of the pitta pulse, the rishis observed *lāvaka, tittiraka* and *kāka gatis. Lāvaka* is a common quail and a lāvaka pulse indicates the possibility of prostatitis in a man or cervicitis in a woman. Tittiraka gati is a partridge pulse, which hops and then stops, showing a sharp spike under the middle finger, indicating a gastric ulcer. *Kāka* means crow and this pulse has a higher spike than tittiraka and denotes an excess pitta disorder in the small intestine (enteritis). This kind of observation is called darshana of the pulse, which leads to *antara darshana*, inner vision or insight. Practicing this, one opens new doors of perception through the tips of the fingers.

The peacock pulse is called *mayūra gati*. It is full and bounding, but the distal phase is spread out like the fan of a peacock. Peacock gati is common in arterial hypertension and it commonly occurs in kapha-pitta people.

Mayūra Gati (Peacock Pulse)

Another interesting dual pulse under the vāta or pitta finger is the camel pulse, which has a hump. Lift the finger and a little notch will be felt, which then drops down. This is called *ushtra* (camel) *gati*. A camel pulse indicates aortic stenosis with thickening or narrowing of the aortic valve.

Ushtra Gati (Camel Pulse)

Under the kapha or ring finger, which generally moves like a swan, one can observe an elephant pulse. The elephant walks slowly and an elephant pulse moves deeply and slowly. Feel the elephant-like movement under the ring finger, letting intuition and awareness work. Before it collapses, the elephant pulse feels like the head of an elephant with a little notch. It is slow, deep and heavy. This pulse is called *gaja gati* and it shows extremely high kapha blocked in the lymphatic tissue. This pulse may also indicate elephantiasis or lymphosarcoma.

Gaja Gati (Elephant Pulse)

Padma Gati (Lotus Pulse)

Also under the kapha finger, one might find *padma gati*, which is a lotus pulse. Just as the lotus moves and floats in the water, the pulse under the finger moves to and fro. The lotus gati is a sacred pulse, indicating that the person is enlightened and the thousand petal lotus of the crown *chakra* is open. The pulse is broad, but moves to and fro, as if there is a constant "so-hum, hum-sa" movement in the breath. This pulse can be present during deep meditation and indicates enlightenment and a blissful state.

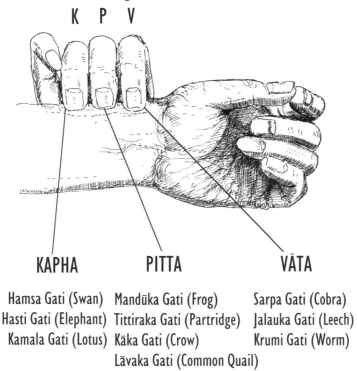

K   P   V

KAPHA   PITTA   VĀTA

KAPHA	PITTA	VĀTA
Hamsa Gati (Swan)	Mandūka Gati (Frog)	Sarpa Gati (Cobra)
Hasti Gati (Elephant)	Tittiraka Gati (Partridge)	Jalauka Gati (Leech)
Kamala Gati (Lotus)	Kāka Gati (Crow)	Krumi Gati (Worm)
	Lāvaka Gati (Common Quail)	

For diagnostic purposes, nādi should not be felt soon after bathing, eating, sex, oil massage, sweating or during thirst, hunger or physical activity.

Feeling the pulse is an art. Awareness should be passive and one should let that awareness act upon the mind. Āyurveda is a subjective as well as an objective science. In recent years, a computerized machine to study the nādi has actually been devised. To use a machine as a diagnostic tool is alright to quantify perception, but to qualify perception requires the sensitivity of the human fingers. Use the tips of the fingers to feel the nature or gati of the pulse and bear in mind the three basic pulses. Certain subtleties about whether the pulse is hot, heavy, light and so forth are difficult to represent graphically. A machine will satisfy some people, but we should program our highly developed human computer, which is our brain, and improve the sensitivity of these beautiful electrodes in the fingertips. When one starts feeling a sarpa, mandūka, hamsa or other gati, a memory is stored in the finger and brain. Through the receptors in the fingertips, one can perceive these characteristics of the different pulses. Once one knows how to perceive, one will begin to gain insight and mastery over the pulse.

Practice these three basic pulses on friends and family and try to become aware of the subtle differences of each individual.

VEGA (RATE)

There are several qualities of the pulse that are relatively gross and easy to read, yet important. One of these qualities, practiced both in Āyurveda and modern allopathic medicine, is *vega*. It means the rate of the pulse, the number of beats per minute. Vega varies due to exercise, anxiety or excitation. To get an accurate resting pulse, take the pulse in the early morning in a restful condition. Vega is normally relatively high in vāta, moderate in pitta and low in kapha. Feel the pulse for one minute and count the number of pulsations.

Vāta   typically around 80-95 beats per minute
Pitta   typically around 65-80 beats per minute
Kapha   typically around 50-65 beats per minute

Vega varies physiologically and according to height and weight. The pulse rate is inversely proportional to height. Tall people generally have slower heart rates and short people have faster heart rates. Children also have higher rates, about 90 to 100 per minute. In older people, the rate is slower. Old age is the age of vāta and the light and rough qualities of vāta weaken the strength of prāna and *vyāna vāyu*, leading to a slow physiological pulse.

Sometimes a slow pulse rate shows slow metabolism. However, a slow pulse is also found in cases of excess kapha, old age and chronic indigestion (which is also *manda agni*). Joggers and other athletes have a slow resting pulse, about 50 to 60, which is healthy. In meditation, the pulse is also slow. However, in the pathological condition of bundle branch block, the rate is slow. Sometimes a *yogi* stops his heart and his metabolism and heart rate become slow. In normal sleep, the pulse rate slows down. A state of anxiety may mask the true rate of the pulse. If someone is feeling your pulse, that thought may enhance the rate of the pulse due to anxiety and stimulation.

Table 4: The Milestones of Age Influencing the Pulse

Infancy/childhood up to 16 years of age	Kapha is predominant in the pulse.
Adult (age 17 - 50)	Pitta is predominant in the pulse.
Adult (age 51 - 70)	Pitta is predominant in the pulse with gradually increasing vāta.
After age 70	Vāta is predominant in the pulse.

The pulse rate becomes high in certain pathological conditions. For example, in anemia, the blood volume is low and the tissues need more oxygen, so the heart increases its rate to provide optimum oxygen to the tissues. Vega is also increased in congestive heart failure, infection, fever, thyrotoxicosis or hyperactive thyroid gland. Thyrotoxicosis is confirmed by reading the pulse while the person is asleep. In this disease, the pulse is high even during deep sleep. All these conditions must be taken into consideration in order to understand whether the vega in an individual is normal or not. However, the moment a doctor with a white coat and stethoscope comes close, a patient's pulse rate increases. Hence it is better to feel the vega at the beginning and end of the examination, in order to get an accurate reading.

When there is an infection, the body sends more blood to the affected area, which increases the pulse rate. There is only one condition where there is infection along with a slow vega and that is typhoid fever. In this condition, a person has a high continuous fever for several days, but the pulse is slow, indicating bradycardia. This is a unique condition. A furry tongue that is centrally coated with red margins, high fever and a slow pulse are the textbook picture of typhoid fever.

The pulse also becomes fast in cases of thyrotoxicosis, anxiety, excitation, exertion, grief, sadness and anger. In thyrotoxicosis the pulse will be fast as long as the toxic goiter is there. Other conditions that create a fast pulse are fever and toxemia.

When some individuals inhale, the pulse rate increases, and on exhalation, the pulse rate slows down. During inhalation the blood rushes from the lungs into the left chambers of the heart, causing the pulse rate to rise. During exhalation, the blood from the right ventricle is pushed into the lungs. This alternation of the pulse rate is called sinus arrhythmia and it is not a pathological condition.

Sinus Arrhythmia Pulse

Remember, the slower the pulse rate, the slower the metabolism, and the faster the pulse rate, the faster the metabolism. Metabolism is governed by *agni*, so when agni is strong, the pulse is relatively fast, light and hot. If agni is slow, the pulse is slow, heavy and cool. In this way, the quality of agni can be understood through a general examination of the pulse.

TĀLA (RHYTHM)

Tāla is rhythm, which is defined as the time interval between two successive uplifts. In the case of a balanced, healthy and normal tāla, the time interval is regular, uninterrupted and rhythmic. This balanced tāla reflects the synchronization of prāna vāyu, vyāna vāyu, avalambaka kapha and sādhaka pitta. When vāta is out of balance, it will create irregularity in the pulse. An irregularly irregular tāla, which means a crazy pulse, involves a disorder of vāta. It may be vāta only, or it could be due to vāta pushing pitta, because vāta is mobile and pitta has a spreading quality. When vāta is pushing pitta, the pulse is fast, feeble and irregularly irregular. This unpredictably irregular pulse is present in atrial flutter with fibrillation.

However, pitta also has a liquid quality, so it can block vāta, causing the pulse to miss a beat. If either pitta or kapha is blocking vāta, the rhythm will be regularly irregular. For example, every third or fourth or seventh beat may be missing, depending on the amount of blockage. Kapha blocking vāta means that, because of some imbalance, the force of kapha dosha is inhibiting the normal activity of vāta. Kapha can block both vāta and pitta, while pitta can also block vāta dosha. On the other hand, vāta can push pitta and kapha, but it cannot block another dosha.

Sometimes a regularly irregular pulse, due to pitta or kapha blocking vāta, indicates an extra systole. This is caused by premature ventricle contraction, or incomplete contraction of the ventricle, resulting in the heart missing a beat. In cases of multiple extra systole, the pulse becomes irregularly irregular.

BALA (FORCE)

Bala is the force or pressure of the pulse. Press the artery with the three fingers. According to Newton's third law of motion, action and reaction are equal and opposite. The amount of force pressing on the blood vessel is also exerted back onto the fingers. That is called bala in Sanskrit. This force is equal to the difference between the systolic and diastolic pressures, which produces a ratio called pulse pressure (PP).

Suppose systolic blood pressure is 120 and diastolic pressure is 70. The difference between these two numbers is 50, which is a normal pulse pressure. In the person with a water hammer pulse, the systolic pressure is around 200 and the diastolic is 30, leading to a PP of about 170, which is extremely high. When the pulse pressure is high, the heart is working under great stress.

In exactly the opposite condition, if the systolic is 70 and the diastolic is 60, the pulse pressure is only 10. This person doesn't receive enough prāna or oxygen to the brain. If pulse pressure is feeble, the person becomes dizzy and may experience transient loss of consciousness or even shock. Bala is generally low in a vāta person, high in a pitta and moderate in a kapha individual.

There is much confusion about bala and how firmly the artery should be pressed in order to feel the force of the pulse. The amount of pressure will vary with the individual, depending upon prakruti and the volume of blood in the radial artery. Quantitatively, high bala can be represented by three plus (+++), low by one plus (+), and moderate by two plus (++). The pluses have a relative meaning here. For instance, a full and bounding pulse is high bala and represented by three pluses. If deep pressure of the finger is necessary in order to stop the artery, that means the force is strong. Moderate pressure indicates the force is moderate. If superficial pressure causes the pulse to disappear, the force is low. The deeper the pressure used to stop the artery, the higher the force. The pulse of an obese person is hard to read because of the adipose tissue, but once you feel it, the bala is usually moderate.

ĀKRUTI (VOLUME AND TENSION)

Ākruti means volume and tension. Volume is experienced as the uplift to the palpating finger. Higher amplitude is higher volume; lower amplitude is lower volume. It is not necessary to depress the radial artery to feel the volume. Just feel the uplift while the fingers rest lightly on the artery. The volume of the pulse corresponds to the systolic blood pressure (the amount of blood that is propelled or pumped out during a ventricular systole). If volume is high, the systolic blood pressure is high. If volume is low, the systolic blood pressure is low. In this way, the Āyurvedic physician reads blood pressure without using a sphygmomanometer.

With high volume, a large amount of blood is propelled through the arterial and venous systems. Pitta has such high volume that it lifts the fingers. Vāta people have low volume and kapha people have moderate volume. The volume is low in congestive heart failure and extremely low blood pressure, such as in cases of anemia and dehydration. In a patient suffering from shock, there is sudden low blood pressure, perspiration and unconsciousness. Pallor, perspiration, pulselessness and falling blood pressure are the cardinal signs of shock.

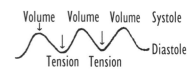

The fullness of the blood vessel depends upon water intake and the quality of *rasa dhātu* as well as the volume of the blood. If a person has good volume of the blood and optimum rasa dhātu, the veins are prominent. Vāta people, who usually do not have sufficient fat, have prominent veins but thin arteries. In contrast, chubby kapha individuals have thin veins but broad arteries. The veins are collapsed and thin in severe anemia, dehydration and blood loss.

In order to feel the volume, press the artery gently and feel the throb against the fingers. An intense throb can be recorded as three plus (+++) volume. If volume is low—one plus (+)—it can barely be felt. This grading system is relative to the individual prakruti. If throbbing is prominent in the middle finger, which is pitta, the volume is good or three plus. That's why a pitta pulse is described as jumping like a frog. If throbbing is felt under the ring finger, which is kapha, it is moderate volume. If throbbing is barely felt under the index finger, vāta, the volume is low.

To describe ākruti fully, one has to determine both volume and tension. Tension is felt by pressing the ring finger to stop the pulsation of the radial artery and then feeling the tension under the middle and index fingers, as if the blood vessel is a rubber tube full of water. Tension is the pressure between two uplifts, which is diastolic pressure. This is the constant pressure of blood in the artery. Although blood is not propelled through the artery, the vessel is never empty. If it were, life would also be empty and the patient would be in shock. Tension is maintained by vyāna vāyu and avalambaka kapha, whereas volume is maintained by prāna vāyu and rañjaka pitta. Rañjaka pitta is hot and it expands the blood vessel, while prāna creates pulsation. Avalambaka kapha, which is present in the heart, maintains the constant pressure of the blood vessels.

We can make some interesting clinical observations regarding volume and tension. If a person with pitta prakruti has a slow pulse rate, such as 55 per minute, but the tension of the pulse is high, he may be taking a beta-blocker for high blood pressure. Beta-blockers can increase kapha dosha in rasa dhātu, which reduces the pulse rate and brings down blood pressure, but may block the bronchial tree by producing congestion.

There is one pulse, called the water hammer pulse in modern medicine, where the volume is high but the tension is low. This pulse has high systolic blood pressure of about 200, but the diastolic reading is only about 30. Such a vast difference between diastolic and systolic blood pressure creates a collapsing pulse. In modern medicine, this pulse is connected to aortic regur-

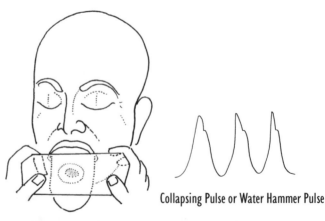

Collapsing Pulse or Water Hammer Pulse

Capillary Pulsation
Press the tongue with a glass slide and an area of blanching will be visible with each systole of the heart. This indicates aortic regurgitation.

gitation. In this condition, the blood goes back from the aorta into the left ventricle, where it vibrates. This is a diastolic murmur that is best heard at the aortic area. If the hand is raised, the throbbing and collapsing nature of the pulse is still felt. This pulse is characteristic of increased pulse pressure, so that even the capillary pulsation is prominent. This condition is further evidenced when pressure on the fingernail causes one portion to be white and one portion to be pink. Because of the increased capillary pulsation, the red part encroaches on the white part. Evidence of capillary pulsation can also be seen on the tongue. Press the tongue with a glass slide. An area of blanching will be visible with each systole of the heart, indicating aortic regurgitation.

TAPAMĀNA (TEMPERATURE)

Tapamāna means temperature. A vāta pulse is cold, pitta is hot and kapha is warm to cool. When vāta dosha is moving through rasa dhātu, the pulse becomes cold. There is a relationship between the gati of the pulse, the wave of the pulse, the temperature of the pulse and the agni or metabolic fire of the individual. When the pulse is cold, fast and light, it means vāta is high and agni is variable—*vishama agni*. When it is hot, sharp and light to the touch, it indicates there is high pitta and *tīkshna* (sharp) *agni*. A heavy, dull pulse shows there is high kapha dosha and manda (slow) agni.

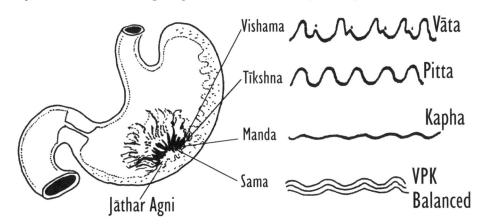

KĀTHINYA (CONSISTENCY OF THE VESSEL WALL)

The consistency of the vessel wall, felt by rolling the artery between the palpating finger and the radial bone, is called *kāthinya*. Palpating in this way reveals whether the vessel wall is thick or thin, elastic or plastic, rigid, hard, or rough.

If vāta is high, its rough and hard qualities cause the blood vessels to also become rough and hard. This may manifest as arteriosclerosis, whereby the blood vessels narrow and there is insufficient blood supply to the brain and other organs. It can also lead to Alzheimer's syndrome, which is a slow death of the brain cells. In high pitta conditions, the blood vessels are elastic but become fragile, creating a tendency to bruise easily. In some individuals, high pitta can cause pressure on the nerves leading to migraine headache. There is also the possibility of capillary hemorrhage, causing the blood vessels to bleed. In high kapha, the blood vessels become broad and thick. The deposition of fat on the wall of the blood vessel (a kapha-like substance) can lead to atheroma, which is one of the causes of hypertension.

These are the seven important conditions to be observed in reading the nādi. Using "Seven Characteristics of the Pulse" on page 13 as a reference, face a partner and read that person's pulse for one minute. The ideal time for an accurate reading of the pulse is early morning on an empty stomach. From the learning point of view, one can read the pulse at any time. Practice reading the pulse on only one hand—the right hand on the male and the left for a female. Facing each other, take the pulse of the subject's left hand with your right hand and vice versa. Never cross the auric field by using the other hand. Feel the pulse from the outer or thumb side of the radial bone. Try to read the vega (speed per minute), gati (manner the pulse moves), tāla (rhythm), bala (force), ākruti (volume and tension), tapamāna (temperature) and kāthinya.

Be clear with feeling. Be vivid with perception. Be honest with pure awareness. Every person should keep a journal of his or her own pulse. It is a meditation. Upon waking, even before passing urine or brushing the teeth, sit quietly on the bed and feel the pulse. Keep a record. Draw a picture. This is the best way to read one's own book, the pulse. Pulse is the vibration of prāna, the pulsation of consciousness under the radial artery. By keeping a record of daily pulse reading, self-knowing unfolds. That is the best way to learn. When one learns how to read one's own pulse, reading the pulses of others will be easy.

Table 5: Examples of Gati and Their Conditions

PULSE	GATI (MOVEMENT)	CONDITIONS
~~	Sarpa gati (Cobra)	Normal vāta pulse
∧∧∧∧∧	Mandūka gati (Frog)	Normal pitta pulse
~~	Hamsa gati (Swan)	Normal kapha pulse
~~	Jalauka gati (Leech)	Arthritis, gout

Table 5: Examples of Gati and Their Conditions

PULSE	GATI (MOVEMENT)	CONDITIONS
	Krumi gati (Worm)	Parasites, worms
	Tittiraka gati (Partridge)	Gastric ulcer, enteritis
	Lāvaka gati (Quail)	Prostatitis, cystitis
	Kāka gati (Crow)	Aortic regurgitation, heart condition
	Mayūra gati (Peacock)	Arterial hypertension, high cholesterol
	Kapota gati (Pigeon)	Bronchial asthma
	Kukkuta gati (Cock)	Diabetes, albuminuria
	Ushtra gati (Camel)	Aortic stenosis, rheumatic valvular heart condition
	Gaja gati (Elephant)	Lymphatic obstruction, solid edema, lymphosarcoma, elephantiasis
	Girija gati (Mountain)	Heart block, bundle branch block
	Vishama gati (Irregular)	Pulsus alternans, atrial fibrillation
	Damaru gati (Vibrating like a drum)	Fatal illness, renal failure, shock
	Pippilika gati (Ants)	Terminal illness
	Padma nādi (Lotus)	Perfect health, enlightenment

सर्प जलौकादिगतिं वदन्ति विबुधाः प्रभञ्जने नाडीम् ।
पित्तेन काक लावक मण्डूकादेस्तथा चपलाम् ॥ ५५ ॥
राजहंस मयूराणां पारावत कपोतयोः ।
कुक्कुटस्य गतिं धत्ते धमनी कफसङ्गिनी ॥ ५६ ॥
यो. र. १

The movements of the cobra and leech are said by the wise to belong to vāta dosha. Those of the crow, quail and frog denote pitta dosha. The swan, peacock, cock and pigeon show kapha dosha in the pulse.

Yoga Ratnakar, 1:55-56

PRAKRUTI AND VIKRUTI
Balance and Imbalance
Levels Seven and One

सर्वं शरीरचरास्तु वातपित्तश्लेष्माणः सर्वस्मिच्छरीरे
कुपिताकुपिताः शुभाशुभानि कुर्वन्ति। ९।
च. सू. २०

*Vāta, pitta and kapha move in the whole body
producing good or ill effects upon the entire
system according to their normal or provoked
states. Their normal state is prakruti and their
abnormal state is vikruti.*

Ca. Sū. 20:9

Vāta, pitta and kapha move in the blood through the rasa and rakta dhātus and it is an interesting fact that the doshas are best felt under specific fingers. We feel the qualities of vāta best under the index finger, because the nerve receptors in that finger best perceive those qualities embraced by vāta—light, subtle, mobile, dry, rough. The same is true for feeling pitta and kapha under the middle and ring fingers, owing to their respective qualities. Vāta is always the distal finger (the finger farthest from the heart) wherever the pulse is palpated, whether it is the wrist, ankle, groin or elsewhere.

I like thinking about all the animals of the pulse being in their homes. When a happy and cheerful cobra is felt under the index finger, a mellow and easy-going frog is felt under the middle finger, and a peacefully swimming swan is under the ring finger, that person is a happy and healthy human being. However, in cases of imbalance, a different animal may be felt under each finger. For instance, a frog may be felt under the index finger, where one should feel a cobra. We can say that the frog is chasing the cobra, which means pitta is blocking vāta. Perhaps under the middle finger one feels a cobra instead of a frog. In that situation, visualize the cobra chasing the frog, which means vāta is pushing pitta. These are only two observations of many that can be made.

Even though the gross manifestations of the three doshas are perceived generally under the index, middle and ring fingers, their subtle qualities are felt under specific areas of each fingertip: at the distal, middle and proximal curvatures.

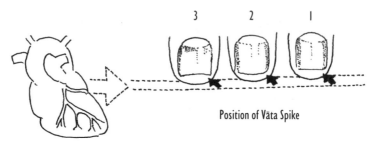

Position of Vāta Spike

The most subtle dosha is vāta, which is light, mobile, subtle and expansive. With very little pressure, the blood flow can be blocked. Even if vāta is partially blocked by the finger, its subtlety will not create a spike at the proximal curvature of each palpating finger. It will easily go through to find space to expand and create a spike at the distal curvature of the fingers, as shown in the picture.

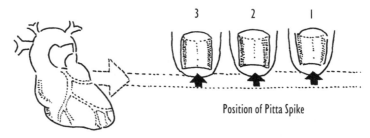

Position of Pitta Spike

Like vāta, pitta is also light, but it is liquid, oily and substantial in nature, whereas vāta is dry and empty. Because of its light and liquid qualities, a pitta spike will be felt at the middle curvature of each of the three fingers.

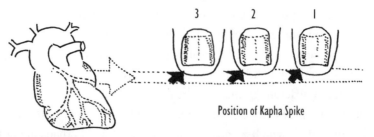

Position of Kapha Spike

Kapha is heavy, oily, static and slow, so it stops at the site on the finger closest to the heart and creates a spike at the proximal curvature of each finger.

In summary, vāta is faster and moves ahead to the distal curvature, pitta is next and moves to a central position next to vāta, while kapha is slow and stops at the proximal curvature. The curvature of the finger is a sensitive instrument, placed directly on the pulse to feel the throb. The art of pulse reading is very subtle and Āyurveda teaches us to be aware of the nature of the body, mind and consciousness of the individual and of the quality of the spikes felt separately under each finger.

The Seven Levels of the Pulse

It is convenient to divide the reading of the radial pulse into seven levels. According to the Āyurvedic system of medicine, there are seven dhātus. If we take a cross-section of any extremity, from the superficial layer to the inner core, the seven dhātus are present. For instance, the superficial layer is *rasa*, the capillary layer is *rakta*, and so forth. Likewise, in the pulse, the superficial level can be called the first level, and if we go to the deepest level, after which the pulse is obliterated, we feel the seventh level. In between the superficial and deep pulse there are another five levels, to make seven in total. As we press down on the radial artery, we can feel the spikes of the pulse change as we move deeper or shallower from one level to another.

These seven levels are not explained in the Āyurvedic texts. There are various systems and methods of reading the pulse and every vaidya has his or her unique technique that has been developed from clinical practice. I respect all those methods. Whatever I say in this book comes from my guru's teaching. Āyurveda has a guru-disciple tradition and I learned about these seven levels from my guru. In modern medicine, the pulse only relates to the cardiovascular system, whereas in Āyurveda, the pulse has a wide range of perception. These seven levels can elaborate in great detail about the prakruti-vikruti paradigm, the state of each subtype of the doshas, the status of prāna, *tejas* and *ojas*, and the condition of the seven bodily tissues. An illustration of all seven levels of the pulse is shown at "The Seven Levels of the Pulse" on page 140. We will now examine each of these levels separately, beginning with the seventh.

THE PRAKRUTI PULSE

At this point, we will bring our attention to prakruti and vikruti and how to read them on the seventh and first levels respectively of the radial pulse. To avoid confusion, be aware that the locations of prakruti and vikruti are referred to in several ways—levels seven and one, deep and superficial levels, the levels of balance and imbalance. Prakruti is one's basic constitution, established at the time of conception, and is read at the seventh or deepest level. Vikruti is our present state and is read on the first or superficial level of the pulse. Āyurveda says that in some individuals, the prakruti may be $V_3P_3K_3$, which means that all doshas are present equally. However, few people are born with this ideal prakruti, called *sama prakruti*. Most people have some combination or variation of the ideal, such as $V_2P_1K_3$ or $V_1P_2K_3$. These numbers indicate the relative ratios of the doshas present in that individual. There is almost always at least one dosha that we can describe as having a level of "3". If there is no "3" in the reading, it indicates the person was born with a depleted dosha, called *dosha kshaya*. *Kshaya* means diminished, deteriorated or deficient.

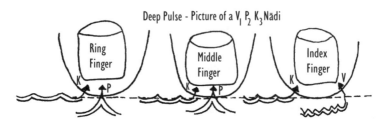

Deep Pulse - Picture of a $V_1 P_2 K_3$ Nādi

When the superficial pulse corresponds to the deep pulse, that person is healthy and balanced. Our present status and our prakruti should be identical. For example, if a person's prakruti at the deep (seventh) level shows $V_2P_3K_1$ and the superficial reading at the first level is the same, that person is balanced. Every individual's balanced state will vary according to his or her constitution.

Some say that the right hand pulse of a man and the left hand pulse of a woman will give the most accurate readings. Others say that both the pulses should be felt, but that it is okay to first master one side. Either way, feel the throb of life under the fingers. Try to evaluate the relative presence of vāta, pitta and kapha. If you feel both arms and the pulses on the right and left sides of the body are just about equal, it indicates that the male and female energies are balanced and vyāna vāyu is moving the doshas equally on both sides. In some individuals, vyāna vāyu pushes a dosha more on one side and that pulse will be more prominent than the other. The pulse may also become feeble on one side, due to previous surgery on the forearm or from a lymph node pressing the main blood vessel.

If pitta is strong in a person's pulse, a spike at the pitta position will be felt under all three fingers, which we describe as $pitta_3$. Likewise, if vāta or kapha is strong, a spike at their positions will be felt under all three fingers, which we describe as $vāta_3$ or $kapha_3$. However if, say, pitta is strong ($pitta_3$) but vāta is feeble, only one vāta spike at the distal position will be noted, which is $vāta_1$. If kapha is relatively strong in that person's pulse, it will create a spike at the proximal position on two fingers. This information shows that person's prakruti is $vāta_1$ $pitta_3$ $kapha_2$, which is abbreviated as $V_1P_3K_2$.

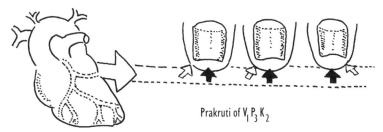

Prakruti of $V_1 P_3 K_2$

There are a number of situations that may lead to an inaccurate reading of the pulse. Sometimes the three fingers are not positioned at the same level. If, say, the ring finger and middle finger press deeply but the index finger is less deep, the reading will not be accurate. In addition, if the index finger is held directly on the radial tubercle, it may not feel any throb. Firstly, individual perception must be ruled out as the cause of an inaccurate reading. Sometimes the appearance of a person can be deceiving. Though the person may look like a healthy, chubby kapha type, the thick subcutaneous fat may cover the true sensation of the pulse. If someone is prematurely born, that person may have a prakruti reading of $V_1 P_1 K_1$. Other factors, such as umbilical strangulation, may also affect the reading. However, these things are not prakruti. They are called vikruti encroaching prakruti and, in these patients, it is difficult to read the real prakruti. In a situation such as this, asking the patient questions will be helpful.

Meditate upon each finger and feel where the spikes are located. We have to be still and observe closely. Pulse reading needs persistent, prolonged practice and it is practice that makes one perfect. This is a technique, but unless it is digested and understood, insight will never come. Insight is a product of repeated practice and through this, the art of pulse reading will develop.

At this point, select someone to practice on. Take their right or left arm and press the radial artery deeply enough to cut off the pulsation. Release slightly, just to the point where the pulsation returns. This is the seventh and deepest level, the level of prakruti. Now feel for the throbs of vāta, pitta and kapha. Count the number of throbs at the vāta site, at the distal curvature of the index, middle and ring fingers. Then feel for the number of pitta throbs in the middle of each of these three fingers. Next, count the number of throbs at the kapha site at the proximal curvature.

THE VIKRUTI PULSE

The section above refers to the seventh level of the pulse, which is the level of prakruti, the physical constitution. Now we will switch our attention to vikruti, the current physical and doshic state. This can be felt at the first level of the pulse. Prakruti is defined as the relative presence of vāta, pitta and kapha at conception. Vikruti is the deviation, either quantitatively or qualitatively, of the doshas from prakruti, the state of the individual's balance. This change can be mild or great, and it can take place over a long period of time or a short one.

Now choose a partner and try to read the prakruti once again. Then release the pressure on the radial artery and come to the superficial pulse, to find out the vikruti. At this level, one again reads vāta, pitta and kapha on the index, middle and ring fingers. Any of the three doshas may show the same reading as for the prakruti pulse or be increased, and occasionally a dosha may be decreased. For example, suppose three people have a prakruti of $V_1P_3K_2$. One person may have P_4 in the vikruti with the other two doshas in the same quantities as in the prakruti, while another might have K_3 in the vikruti and the other two doshas the same, and a third person could have all three doshas at the same levels as the prakruti. In other words, at the superficial level, one, two or even all three doshas can be increased above their prakruti levels or may show a stronger qualitative presence.

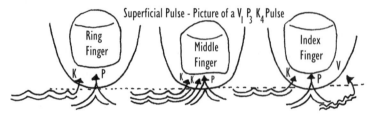

Superficial Pulse - Picture of a $V_1 P_3 K_4$ Pulse

Remember the earlier discussion (*see* "General Characteristics of Vāta, Pitta and Kapha Pulses" on page 11) about the characteristics of the spike. When checking the vikruti pulse at the superficial level, the quality of the spike is particularly important for determining the state of imbalance. Spikes at the kapha position may be felt on one, two, or all three fingers, but there may also be an extra kapha spike in the vāta or pitta region of a finger. That's why kapha can be counted as four in the case of someone with a vikruti of, say, $V_1P_3K_4$. The same is also true for vāta and pitta doshas. For instance, there may be an extra vāta spike, which is quavery, in the superficial pulse either under the ring or middle finger. If vāta appears under the middle finger at the pitta site, it means that vāta is pushing pitta in the vikruti. If it appears under the ring finger at the kapha site, it indicates vāta pushing kapha.

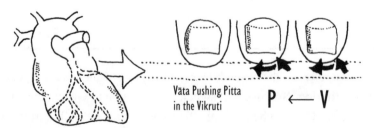

Vāta Pushing Pitta in the Vikruti $P \leftarrow V$

In terms of how to quantify the vikruti pulse, we can say that an extra spike at the dosha's own site is counted as an extra V_1, P_1 or K_1, whereas an extra spike at another dosha's site is counted as an extra $V_{0.5}$, $P_{0.5}$ or $K_{0.5}$. Note that half a dosha will never be read in the prakruti, only in the vikruti. One needs to pay close attention to the doshic qualities of the spikes.

There are many subtleties in the pulse. A description of a tree is not the tree. Likewise, a description of a pulse is not the pulse itself. We are trying to bring subjective experience to the objective level, which is most difficult. There are many things to be taken into consideration. The quality of the spike and sensitivity of the fingers should be observed. Don't accept only what is written here; believe in your own perception. The pulse reading depends upon subjective observation and the quality of perception. Many times, when reading the pulse of a subject, we will observe that two examiners arrive at different diagnoses from one another. It is a matter of perception and experience.

When I read the pulse, I do so-hum meditation. So-hum is a great *mantra*. My guru told me to inhale "so" and exhale "hum" and go into the space between "so" and "hum", and between "hum" and "so." Breathe in "so" and take the breath deep inside behind the belly button with the inhalation. Stay a moment in that pause. "Hum" goes out with the breath to about nine inches away from the nostrils, where there is a second pause. Feel the pulse during that pause. Reading the pulse is a great meditation. Start reading the pulse by doing so-hum meditation for a few minutes and then bow to the patient. Reading the pulse is like reading that person's book. "Look" into the third eye of the subject, feel the pulse, and then close the eyes and meditate with so-hum breath. Stay either in the outer or inner pause, feeling the pulse and finding the position of the spikes.

The Āyurvedic art of learning is more than just mechanical or technical. Technique is a small part, but sensitive perception and awareness are most important. For example, when you and I look at an object, we look from different angles. When our perception is on the same level, at the same time, with the same intensity and on the same platform, we will perceive the same object and our observations will go hand in hand. However, there will still be personal differences. That doesn't mean that one person is wrong, but in the case of reading the pulse, it could mean that each person may be on a different level. For instance, the prakruti pulse is the seventh level and if one examiner feels the sixth level, the readings will be different. So even though there are genuine differences of perception, it is also possible that varied readings may be caused by the assessment of different levels of the pulse.

3

ORGAN PULSES
Levels Seven and One

The organ pulses are also found on the first and seventh levels, which are the superficial and deep pulses. Hollow organs are located on the superficial level and solid or semi-solid organs are felt at the deep level. Refer to the table on the next page for the locations of each organ.

To take this pulse, use one finger at a time and feel the throbbing. In a healthy condition, the strength of the pulse should be equal between the superficial and deep pulses of each finger. However, if an organ is weak, a feeble throb will be felt in the pulse under the related finger. For instance, suppose the colon is weak. In that case, under the index finger on the right hand side of the subject, a weaker spike will be felt on the superficial pulse than on the deep pulse. Always compare the force (bala) of the superficial and deep pulses under the same finger. Ideally, the two pulses have the same force, indicating they are working cooperatively. However one may be stronger than the other. Record the reading for each organ. The stronger pulse can be represented by a plus (+) and a weaker pulse by a minus (-).

Āyurvedic literature states that the liver and spleen are the root of *rakta vaha srotas*, the hematopoietic system. It is my observation that the liver pulse is situated on the right side of the subject and the spleen pulse on the left. In the Chinese system, the liver and gallbladder are on the left wrist of the subject and the stomach and spleen on the right. In Āyurvedic texts, there is no mention about specifically reading the organs through the pulse. However, the organs are included in the concept of *srotāmsi* (bodily channels).

Now choose a partner and read the status of each organ pulse. With the aid of the diagrams on the next two pages, try to feel the relative strength of the superficial and deep pulses under each finger. Find out if any organs are weak by feeling the force of the pulse's throbbing. If the throbbing is strong, the strength of the organ is good and you can classify that as a plus. If the throbbing is feeble, the strength is weak, and it can be classified as a minus.

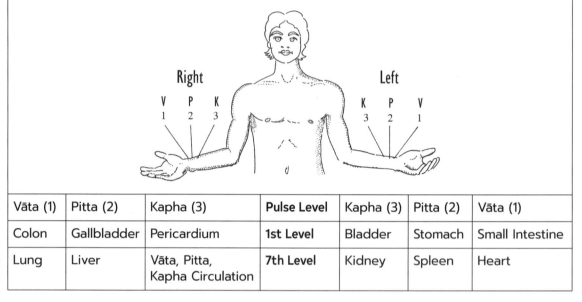

Vāta (1)	Pitta (2)	Kapha (3)	Pulse Level	Kapha (3)	Pitta (2)	Vāta (1)
Colon	Gallbladder	Pericardium	**1st Level**	Bladder	Stomach	Small Intestine
Lung	Liver	Vāta, Pitta, Kapha Circulation	**7th Level**	Kidney	Spleen	Heart

Some people may have very strong deep organs, which means they have a strong constitution. In some the hollow organs are weak, which means their vikruti is more prevalent in the superficial organs. If the pulse of a deep organ is weak, it may mean that a dosha has gone deep into the prakruti and is affecting that organ.

Āyurveda talks about the concept of a *khavaigunya* or defective space within the body. This defective or weak space may be in an organ, *srotas* (system), localized area, dhātu (tissue), etc., resulting from many possible factors—for example, traumas, genetic inheritance, wrong diet or lifestyle. Once the space is weakened, a circulating aggravated dosha (*prasara* stage in *samprāpti*) may begin to accumulate there and initiate pathological changes.

The strength of an organ may also be depleted due to an accumulation of *āma* or because of low agni in that particular organ. This can also be felt as a feeble organ pulse. The organ pulse may become feeble without indicating any doshic spike. This shows that there is weakness, khavaigunya, in that organ, but the dosha has not yet lodged there and created a pathological condition. If this condition is not treated, any aggravated dosha may lodge in the organ to create pathological changes, at which point the doshic spike develops.

Generally, observation shows that in people who have more solar or male energy—even women can be more masculine and sometimes aggressive—the organs are more activated during the daytime. In those with lunar or female-dominant energy, the organs become active during the night. When female energy in a man becomes active, he becomes more compassionate, loving and emotional.

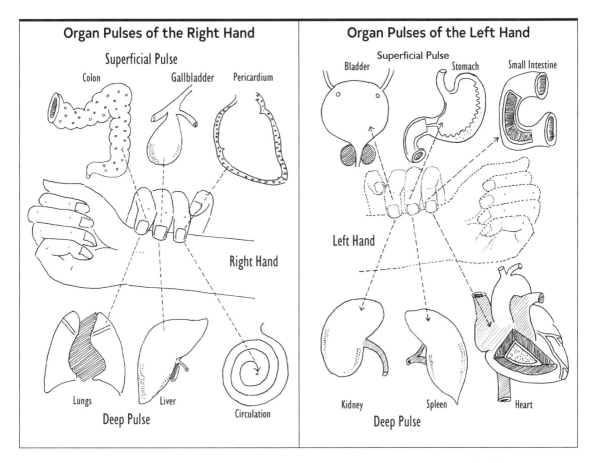

If any organ is removed surgically, that organ's pulse will be feeble. If the gallbladder is removed, the gallbladder pulse will be weak. If a lobe of a lung is removed, the lung pulse will be feeble. If there is a transplanted organ, the transplanted organ pulse may also be feeble or absent, because that organ doesn't belong to the person's prakruti. Ideally it is better to receive an organ from someone of the same prakruti. If the prakruti is quite different, that will increase the likelihood of rejection of the transplanted organ.

Each organ stores memory in its connective tissue. Memory is stored not only in the brain but also in the heart, liver and other organs. Our entire body is a memory body. Our entire body is an emotional body. When an organ is transplanted from one body into another, this stored memory goes with the organ and becomes a part of the recipient's memory.

Colon

The superficial pulse under the index finger on the right side of the subject corresponds to the colon. If a strong spike is felt, the colon is strong. If the organ becomes weak there will be a feeble pulse. If the colon pulse is feeble and throbbing is felt at the kapha location, there is a possibility of excess mucus, parasites, amebae or some tumor in the colon. When there is chronic amebiasis, which is a kapha disorder in which the body walls off the infection, the mucous membrane rolls and creates a lump called an ameboma, which is a kapha type of tumor.

If the colon pulse is weak with a throb at the pitta area, there may be excess pitta in the colon causing colitis, diverticulitis, chronic diarrhea or dysentery, appendicitis, pitta-type hemorrhoids or bleeding polyps. If the spike is at the vāta area and the colon pulse is low, the person may have chronic constipation, gases in the colon or gulma. Kapha-type *gulma* (tumor) is an ameboma, vāta-type gulma is diverticulosis and pitta-type gulma is diverticulitis and polyp. A polyp may be mucus or it may be a ruptured blood vessel causing profuse bleeding due to a pitta disorder.

The lungs and colon are linked as important organs related to *prāna vaha srotas*. The qualities of vāta are cold, dry, light, mobile and subtle and these can affect the colon. For example, the mobile quality can carry excess pitta from the small intestines or gallbladder into the colon, causing colitis. In such a case, the colon pulse will be weak and there will be an extra vāta spike in the pitta position on the index finger of the right hand. Making this type of diagnosis is a complicated process with many subtleties.

When vāta is pushing pitta, pitta becomes aggravated and may manifest in the colon or some other organ, rather than its home in the small intestine. In such a case, pitta is innocent and vāta dosha is the problem. It is samāna vāyu that pushes pāchaka pitta into the colon, or else apāna vāyu can pull pāchaka pitta. Pitta, being hot, can then inflame the colon and there may be rectal bleeding or a burning anus. In symptomatology, vāta symptoms appear first—constipation, bloating, indigestion, burping, insomnia and low agni. Then later, the subject gets pitta symptoms and the pulse shows a typical vāta pushing pitta spike. Note that one should firstly treat the symptoms with the most significant manifestations. If the person is bleeding from the rectum and has a burning colon, don't treat vāta, even though it is the cause. Instead, treat pitta dosha first.

A vāta pushing pitta condition will manifest symptoms according to the site of kha-vaigunya. Suppose apāna vāyu is out of balance and there are toxins in the liver with aggravated rañjaka pitta. With this condition vāta can easily pull rañjaka pitta into the colon, leading to dark yellow or green stools. But suppose the person frequently eats black beans, cayenne pepper, curry pepper, chili pepper and drinks alcohol, causing one's pāchaka pitta to be imbalanced. Then udāna vāyu will push pāchaka pitta upward and create nausea and vomiting. The subtype of vāta involved in the imbalance depends upon the location of the khavaigunya. In a way, there is an affinity between the aggravated sub-dosha and the khavaigunya. *Apāna* pulls down, *udāna* pushes upward and *vyāna* circulates. To assess which subtype is involved, one can simply look at the symptoms. If a person has a bleeding rectum, burning urethra, or vaginal bleeding along with some vāta symptoms, it denotes vāta pushing or pulling pitta. All of the above mentioned cases show apāna vāyu pulling pitta down. Suppose vyāna vāyu is aggravated and pushes rañjaka pitta into the skin, creating hives, rash and acne or bleeding under the skin. When udāna vāyu is pushing pitta upward, there is nausea, vomiting, bloodshot eyes and hot flashes. Wherever pitta is pulled or pushed, there it will create inflammatory changes leading to infection of the affected organs.

Feeble Colon Pulse (Superficial) under the Index Finger on the Right Side

With kapha spike indicates:
Mucus in the colon
Parasites
Amebiasis
Cystic tumor
Ameboma

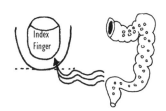

With pitta spike denotes:
Excess pitta in the colon
Colitis
Diverticulitis
Dysentery
Appendicitis
Hemorrhoids
Polyps
Irritable bowel syndrome

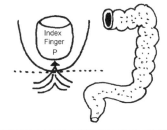

With vāta spike shows:
Excess vāta in the colon
Gases
Constipation
Diverticulosis
Fissure
Fistula

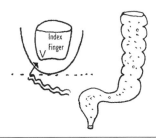

Qualities must also be assessed to understand the type of disorder that may be manifesting as a result of the doshic infiltration of the organ. Some examples of how specific diseases manifest in the colon pulse are given here:

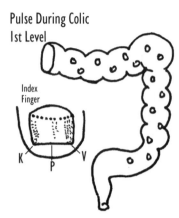

Pulse During Colic
1st Level

Index
Finger

K   P   V

Pakvāshaya Shūla (Colic). During pain due to colic, the pulse becomes feeble and fast at the colon pulse site. The spike is quick, crooked and cold to the touch if it is vāta colic due to spasm. If the spike is at the pitta site and the pulse is sharp, heaving and jerky, it is pitta pain and may be due to acute infection or inflammation which manifests as diarrhea, dysentery or irritable bowel syndrome. On the other hand, if the spike is at the kapha site and the pulse is slow, full, wavy and heavy, it denotes kapha pain due to congestion, amebiasis, giardiasis or worms. If the colon pulse simultaneously shows vāta, pitta and kapha, this may indicate malignant changes, a tridoshic disorder.

Vāta Gulma (Diverticulosis). The colon pulse is feeble and hollow, and it shows a vāta spike. This is a sign of high vāta in the colon. This pulse diagnosis will need to be correlated to other symptoms of diverticulosis, as this pulse can also indicate bloating or constipation. Apāna vāyu creates a cul-de-sac in the colon, causing hardened feces to be trapped.

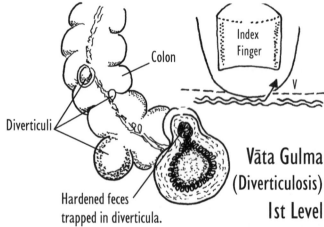

Colon

Index
Finger

V

Diverticuli

Hardened feces
trapped in diverticula.

Vāta Gulma
(Diverticulosis)
1st Level

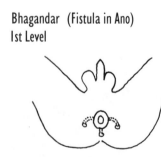

Bhagandar (Fistula in Ano)
1st Level

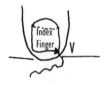

Index
Finger   V

Bhagandar (Anal Fistula). In cases of anal fistula, the colon pulse shows a vāta spike. The pulse is feeble, slippery and depressed.

Lungs

The deep pulse under the index finger on the right side of the subject is related to the lungs. If the lung pulse is feeble with throbbing under the kapha position, there is the possibility of pulmonary congestion, upper respiratory congestion or descending infection. There may be a history of pneumonia, bronchiectasis or pleurisy with effusion. Postnasal drip travels from the nose, into the throat, the trachea and then into the lungs. Kapha is heavy and moves downward. *Bodhaka kapha* (in the mouth) enters tarpaka kapha (in the sinuses) and moves down into avalambaka kapha which is located in the lungs. With excess kapha, the lungs become too damp and cold. Fungus may also enter the lungs, creating fungal infection. If a person is allergic to mold, damp and cold weather, there is excess kapha in the lungs. In addition, when there is surplus kapha in the lungs, a person may get hay fever or pollen allergy during the spring, that is, kapha season.

Feeble Lung Pulse (Deep) under the Index Finger on the Right Side

With kapha spike indicates:
Pulmonary congestion
Hay fever
Upper respiratory congestion
Pneumonia with consolidation
Bronchitis
Asthma
Pleurisy

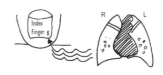

With pitta spike denotes:
Bacterial infection
Tracheitis
Bronchitis
Inflammation
Bleeding in the lungs
Alveolitis

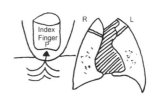

With vāta spike shows:
Cold, dry lungs
Dry pleurisy
Respiratory allergy
Wheezing
Dry cough
Hoarseness of voice
Emphysema

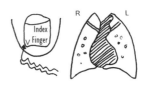

If pitta is involved in problems of the lungs, the spike will be at the middle position of the index finger, indicating a possibility of bacterial infection. Pitta can create bronchitis, tracheitis, bronchiolitis, alveolitis or pleuritis. Perhaps pitta will create a condition of inflamed mucous membranes, indicating too much heat in the lungs. Excess pitta may cause chemical sensitivity. On the emotional level, the lungs are the seat of unresolved grief and sadness, which may create a khavaigunya in the lungs.

Tamaka Svāsa (Emphysema and Asthma). Emphysema is a chronic vāta disorder in which the alveoli, the tiny air sacs in the lungs, become over-inflated with the trapped air of prāna. There are three types of asthma—vāta, pitta and kapha. In vāta asthma there is dry wheezing, a pollen allergy, or spasm to the bronchial tree. A feeble vāta spike will be felt in the lung pulse. Pitta asthma manifests as asthmatic bronchitis. Kapha asthma is more allergy-oriented, a descending infection from the nose leading to cold, cough and wheezing. A kapha spike also shows pneumonia, bronchiectasis or pulmonary congestion, which is a condition of dilation of the bronchi with accumulated mucus.

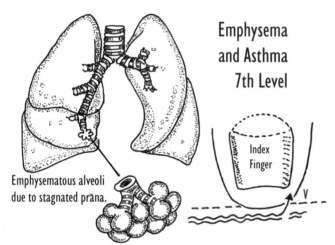

Emphysema
and Asthma
7th Level

Index
Finger

Emphysematous alveoli
due to stagnated prāna.

Rāja Yakshmā (Pulmonary Tuberculosis or Consumption). If the lung pulse feels jerky, feeble and slow, it indicates low prāna in the lungs. If the patient has pulmonary tuberculosis, the lung pulse shows kapha at one moment, pitta at the second moment, and then vāta, which means three doshas are entering the lungs. With tridoshic involvement the person may develop bronchogenic carcinoma. In tuberculosis there is low grade fever, evening rise of temperature, and nocturnal perspiration with extremely low ojas. These signs are absent in carcinoma. In this way one can distinguish between the two disorders and come to a conclusion about the assessment.

Tuberculosis
7th Level

Index
Finger

Vata

Kāsa (Cough). If the lung pulse becomes feeble and slow and beats at the kapha site, it denotes cough due to bronchial congestion. For pitta pushing kapha in the lungs, drink one cup of ginger and licorice tea with 10 drops of Mahānārāyana Oil, an Āyurvedic medicated oil. Take this tea, sip by sip, to release the green mucus. Āyurveda is very specific. It doesn't treat the organ alone but it deals with the root causative dosha. However, while treating the dosha, think about which organ is involved. When there is pitta pushing kapha in the lungs, there is specific management for that condition.

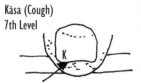

Kāsa (Cough)
7th Level

Vāta involvement in the lungs creates a spike at the distal position of the index finger. A feeble pulse at this position may indicate respiratory allergy, wheezing, dry

cough or hoarseness of voice. Vāta in the lungs can cause inflation, an unnatural disten-
tion with air. This phenomenon is called emphysema. The over-inflated alveoli rupture,
resulting in diminished air entry and air hunger.

Gallbladder

The superficial pulse of the middle finger on the subject's right side is connected to the
gallbladder. A feeble pulse at the kapha site indicates excess kapha in the gallbladder
which will make the gallbladder sluggish, creating thick bile and possibly gallstones.
Because of excess kapha in the gallbladder, the person becomes sensitive to fatty fried
food. Even the fat from peanut butter may create a headache and a dull aching pain in
the right hypochondriac region (liver area).

A feeble gallbladder spike at the pitta location indicates excess pitta in the gallbladder. This may create cholecystitis, an inflamed gallbladder. The person has pain and ten-
derness and pressure put on the gallbladder causes the person to flinch. High pitta in the
gallbladder may also create acid indigestion and lead to duodenal ulcer. Pitta here will
create a sense of tightness in the mid-back.

Feeble Gallbladder Pulse (Superficial) under the Middle Finger on the Right Side

With kapha spike indicates:
Sluggish gallbladder
Excess kapha in gallbladder
Gallstones
Obstructive jaundice

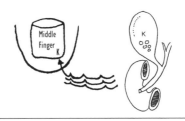

With pitta spike denotes:
Cholecystitis
Over-secretion of bile
Acid indigestion
Duodenal ulcer
Nausea
Vomiting

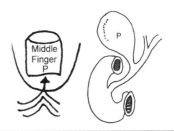

With vāta spike shows:
Insufficient bile
Removal of gallbladder
Spasm of gallbladder
Deformed gallbladder

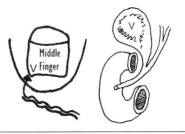

Vāta in the gallbladder will create tightness in the neck and shoulders due to referred pain from the gallbladder. If the gallbladder pulse is feeble with a spike at vāta, the gallbladder has insufficient bile.

When gallstones are present, the spike may be at the kapha site or at the pitta site, because both are involved in this condition. Sometimes just by feeling the pulse one can tell about the presence of gallstones, which can be verified through x-ray. X-ray can show calcified stones, but if the stones are soft, the x-ray will pass through them without casting a shadow on the film. However, soft stones can be detected with ultrasound. Sometimes the spike will be felt in between pitta and kapha, indicating hepatic conges-tion. Though stones are formed in the gallbladder and the changes can be felt in the gall-bladder superficial pulse, the deep liver pulse also shows doshic changes. Even in cholecystitis, which is inflammation of the gallbladder, the pathology of the stone begins in the liver. The bile becomes thick and oily due to excess kapha which then accumulates in the gallbladder, causing crystallization of bile that leads to soft stones. Later these stones become calcified and hard.

Liver

The deep pulse under the middle finger on the right radial pulse of the subject is associ-ated with the liver. A feeble liver pulse with a spike at kapha indicates excess kapha which can create fatty degenerative changes. The liver becomes enlarged and such a liver cannot digest fatty fried food. When there is excess kapha in the liver, it may denote serum hepatitis where the virus lives in the kapha molecules of body fluid, e.g., serum, saliva and semen. The person may get hepatitis B which can become hepatitis C due to post-transfusion complications, leading to cirrhotic changes. Cirrhotic changes in the liver are a tridoshic disorder. Cirrhosis of the liver is the death of liver cells but, if detected in the early stages of cirrhosis, the liver can be regenerated. Excess kapha in the liver can cause lipomas, which are fatty tumors, and can also create high cholesterol. The liver synthesizes cholesterol into testosterone, so a person with excess kapha in the liver is bound to have low libido. Rañjaka pitta contains *bhūta agni* which nourishes *dhātu agni*. The strength of *shukra agni* depends upon the energy of the bhūta agni of the liver. One of the causes of obesity is excess kapha in the liver. Obesity, hyperten-sion, high cholesterol and low libido go together.

Excess pitta in the liver can aggravate rañjaka pitta, leading to hepatitis A (infec-tious hepatitis) and jaundice. It may create bleeding tendencies, such as bleeding gums, piles, bloodshot eyes or capillary hemorrhages that cause a person to bruise easily. High pitta in the liver may also make the person emotionally judgmental, angry and critical indicating deep-seated unresolved anger, envy and hatred stored in the liver. In the case of hepatitis A or B, the liver pulse will be feeble, but the spike will show pitta, because hepatitis is a rañjaka pitta disorder. In addition, excess pitta in the liver may lead to chronic fatigue syndrome and mononucleosis, causing a person to feel tired and exhausted. This condition can be treated with several pitta-pacifying Āyurvedic herbs. If the liver enzymes SGOT and SGPT in a blood test are elevated, pitta in the liver is high.

If these enzyme levels are low in the blood, it may be a sign of high vāta. When vāta is high, pitta may be suppressed and liver enzymes may be diminished. With these conditions, the high vāta may create cirrhotic changes. Due to vāta, the liver cells shrink and become dry. Because of the rough quality of vāta, the form of the liver cells is disturbed. The result is increased hepatic pressure which leads to portal hypertension. This condition will push pitta. Vāta pushing pitta in the hematopoietic system may cause bleeding, so vāta in the liver is a serious condition, which is denoted by a vāta spike with a weak liver pulse.

Feeble Liver Pulse (Deep) under the Middle Finger on the Right Side

With kapha spike indicates:
Fatty, degenerative changes
Enlarged liver (hepatomegaly)
Hepatitis B (serum hepatitis)
Multiple lipomas
High cholesterol
Obesity
Hypertension
Low libido

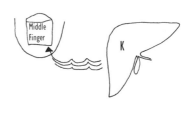

With pitta spike denotes:
Hepatitis A (infectious hepatitis)
Jaundice
Mononucleosis
Hemorrhagic condition
Deep-seated anger, hate
Chronic fatigue syndrome
Copper toxicity

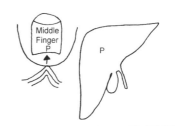

With vāta spike shows:
Suppressed liver enzymes
Shrinking of the liver cells
Cirrhotic changes
Hepatitis C (post-transfusional)
Portal hypertension

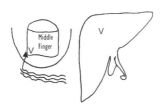

Rañjaka pitta is necessary for coloring rasa dhātu by producing red blood cells, and excess pitta in the liver can affect the production of red blood cells and may create sickle cell, aplastic or megaloblastic anemia as per the conditions. The fire component of rañjaka pitta, which is bhūta agni, affects *rakta dhātu agni* and may result in these anomalies.

Lyme disease is transmitted by the deer tick and the venom of this tick is highly pit-tagenic. If a person is bitten by one of these small ticks, the bhrājaka pitta under the skin is disturbed and affects rañjaka pitta in the blood, which in turn disturbs the rañjaka pitta in the liver and rakta dhātu, producing recurrent inflammatory disorders, accompanied by distinctive skin lesions, erythremia, migraines, polyarthritis and involvement of the heart and nervous system. So Lyme disease increases pitta in the liver. This excess pitta can affect rañjaka pitta and rakta dhātu. The person may get aplastic anemia, which means the red blood cells are not well formed. The liver maintains the consistency of the blood, and coagulation and bleeding time depend entirely upon its function. Therefore, Āyurveda treats the liver in order to regulate the normal function of rakta vaha srotas.

The liver and spleen are the seat of rañjaka pitta and rakta vaha srotas, so the agni (fire) which is present in the liver can regulate the function of the spleen. The spleen is a reservoir of blood. The malarial parasite lodges in the spleen causing the spleen to become enlarged. When the spleen is enlarged, rañjaka pitta is affected, which also affects bhūta agni in the liver. This condition diminishes the effectiveness of the immune system. All these conditions can produce a pitta spike with a feeble liver pulse.

Kāmala (Jaundice). In jaundice, or *kāmala*, the liver pulse becomes feeble at the pitta site and the spike moves like an exhausted frog. A vāta spike in the liver pulse may indicate cirrhotic changes. Cirrhosis is hardening of the liver, the death of the liver cells. A vāta spike also shows hepatitis C, which may lead to cirrhotic changes or cancer of the liver.

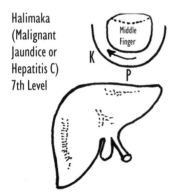

Halimaka (Malignant Jaundice or Hepatitis C) 7th Level

Kāmala (Jaundice)

Halimaka (Malignant Jaundice or Hepatitis C). If, on the liver pulse, there is a pitta spike that moves toward the kapha site (as shown in the diagram) and the pulse is low, tremulous and deep-seated, chronic hepatitis C may manifest as malignant jaundice.

Pericardium

The pericardium has a special pulse under the ring finger at the superficial level on the right hand side of the subject. *Hridaya dhārā kalā* means the membranous structure around the heart. There are two hridaya dhārā kalās, the parietal pericardium and the visceral pericardium. Within the space of the pericardium there is also a fluid, which is one of the components of avalambaka kapha. The pericardium is a membranous structure which is supported by avalambaka kapha. The myocardium, the muscles of the heart and the endocardium, the inner lining of the heart, are also hridaya dhārā kalā. Avalambaka kapha is present in the lungs, the bronchi and bronchioles, and it supports the lungs. The alveoli are constantly breathing air, day in and day out, and the presence of avalambaka kapha in the lungs prevents drying of lung tissue.

उरः स्थः स त्रिकस्य स्ववीर्यतः ।
हृदयस्यान्नवीर्याच्च तत्स्थ एवाम्बुकर्मणा ॥ १५ ॥
कफधाम्नां च शोषाणां यत्करोत्यवलम्बनम् ।
अतोऽवलम्बकः श्लेष्मा
वा. सू. १२

Through its energy flow, avalambaka kapha goes to the neck, arms and sacrum where it supports all kapha systems via circulation through the heart.

Asht. Hrud. Sū. 12:15

Avalambaka kapha enters into rasa and rakta dhātus. Through its energy flow, it goes to the neck, arms and sacrum where it supports all kapha systems via circulation through the heart. Kledaka kapha enters only into rasa dhātu. It lubricates all kapha systems, while avalambaka kapha supports all kapha systems. The pericardium moves with the heart and, in this movement, the pericardium, the hridaya dhārā kalā, generates electricity. That electrical potential, the electrical impulse, is carried through the mucous membrane of the blood vessels. In the same way, around the nerve cells there is a membranous structure that generates electricity and that electricity is carried under the skin.

Feeble Pericardium Pulse (Superficial) under the Ring Finger on the Right Side

With kapha spike indicates:
Attachment
Greed
Possessiveness
Pericardial effusion

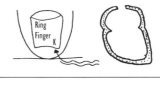

With pitta spike denotes:
Pericarditis
Anger
Hate
Not being loved
Rejection

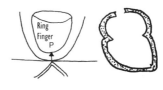

With vāta spike shows:
Anxiety
Fear
Grief
Sadness
Constrictive pericarditis

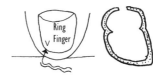

During sex a surplus amount of electricity is generated, causing the heart to beat fast. Therefore, excessive sexual activity can deplete the energy of the pericardium. The electrical energy created by hridaya dhārā kalā can also be influenced by any hot food taken in excess which can activate pericardial movements, stimulate circulation and cause heartburn and irritation.

If the pericardial pulse is feeble with a spike at the kapha curvature, there is a possibility of congestion in the pericardium which may lead to avalambaka kapha blocking prāna, creating bradycardia or slow heart rate. If the right side of the pericardium is blocked, it will create right bundle branch block and left bundle branch block—RBBB and LBBB. Emotionally, the pericardium is related to unresolved, deep-seated attachment and unresolved grief. In extreme emotional conditions, kapha is provoked, leading to a feeble pericardial pulse and pericardial congestion.

If the pericardial pulse is feeble and the spike is felt at the pitta site, there is pericardial inflammation, pericarditis and non-inflammatory burning sensation. When one eats hot foods like cayenne pepper, curry pepper and chili pepper and gets a burning sensation, it is called a non-inflammatory burning sensation. There is also a non-inflammatory burning sensation of the urethra, which is pitta. Pericardial congestion, non-inflammatory heartburn, is common in gastritis and hyperacidity. Because of the nerve connection, a burning sensation in the stomach creates referred pain in the heart area. Therefore, excess pitta can create pericardial congestion and heartburn. Emotionally there may be unresolved anger, hatred and a feeling of rejection stuck in the heart and the pericardium.

Relationship has such a great value. It is responsibility and commitment. But these days people have lost the true significance of relationship. A relationship in turmoil affects the pericardium and a feeling of rejection may lead to constrictive pericarditis, which may be associated with tuberculosis in the long term.

Now we will consider vāta. When the pericardial pulse is feeble with a spike at the distal curvature, the site of vāta, it may indicate multiple extra systole. The pulse will be irregular with a possibility of atrial flutter with fibrillation. Premature ventricle systole may also be due to aggravation of vāta in the pericardium. A vāta spike in the pericardial pulse can denote deep-seated fear, insecurity and loneliness. Thus, Āyurveda uses the pericardial pulse to understand the emotional status of the subject.

Circulation

The deep pulse on the ring finger of the subject's right hand corresponds to the circulation. It is fascinating that the heart, such a small organ, creates a wave that doesn't die. The pulsation of this wave goes to the tips of the fingers and toes. This capability is due to the functional integration of vāta, pitta and kapha. Vāta is expansive and clear. Pitta is hot (*ushna*), sharp (*tīkshna*), liquid (*drava*) and flowing (*sara*). Kapha is slow (*manda*), heavy (*guru*) and oily (*snigdha*). The common factor between vāta and pitta is light, between vāta and kapha is cold and between kapha and pitta is oily. Heat expands and cold contracts. The light quality creates upward movement and the heavy quality creates downward movement. These combined qualities of three doshas help to carry the pulsations of the heart as a wave that is moved through the pulse to the tips of the fingers and toes. All of this is the functional integration of tridosha. The impulse that takes place at the heart is carried throughout the body by vyāna vāyu. Vyāna vāyu, rañjaka pitta and kledaka kapha move throughout the body. Though rañjaka pitta is in the liver, it enters into the blood and makes the blood hot. If the blood supply to an organ is cut off, that organ becomes cold because of insufficient rañjaka agni.

संतत्या भोज्य धातूनां परिवृत्तस्तु चक्रवत् ॥ २१ ॥
च. चि. १५

The food precursors are moving throughout the body like a wheel through rasa and rakta.

Ca. Ch. 15:21

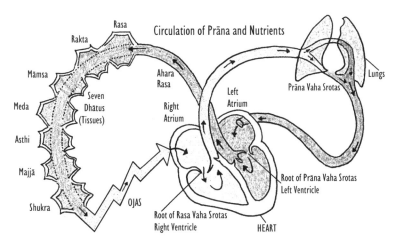

The left chambers of the heart are the root of prāna vaha srotas which circulates the life energy (prāna) to all seven tissues. The right chambers of the heart are the root of rasa vaha srotas which circulates the food nutrients, prāna, tejas and ojas to all seven dhātus with the functional integrity of prāna vāyu, vyāna vāyu, avalambaka kapha and sādhaka pitta in the heart.

We have three diaphragms—the pelvic, abdominal thoracic and cerebral. The cerebral diaphragm supports the brain. With gentle movement it acts as a pump. The plates of the skull move slightly. In craniosacral work, the little movements of the bones of the skull expand prāna vāyu, alter the state of consciousness and bring functional integrity in the organs. There is a thick network of blood vessels in the brain. Some people have a cold scalp, which means their prāna is weak, because the cerebral diaphragm doesn't move properly. This lack of prāna may cause dizziness or ringing in the ear.

The abdominal thoracic diaphragm moves the lungs. On inhalation more blood rushes from the lungs into the left chamber of the heart. On exhalation more blood from the right chamber goes into the lungs. So inhalation and exhalation regulate circulation. The abdominal thoracic diaphragm brings more blood to the arms. Therefore, cold hands mean poor circulation from incomplete diaphragmatic breathing.

The pelvic diaphragm is governed by apāna vāyu and it regulates the circulation in the lower extremities. On squatting, the pelvic muscles contract and the stool is easily passed. Cold legs indicate weak apāna; cold hands, weak samāna; cold scalp, weak prāna. The concept of circulation in Āyurveda is very interesting. Though vyāna vāyu is responsible for circulation, it is influenced by prāna, samāna and apāna respectively, which can be detected at the seventh level of the pulse under the ring finger.

Vyāna vāyu circulates throughout the body. Vyāna goes down with the help of apāna and moves up with the help of udāna. These movements are nothing but circulation. That is why in the Chinese system circulation is called Triple Heater. What is Triple Heater? Triple Heater is vāta, pitta and kapha with functional integration. When the Chinese system speaks about Triple Heater, in the Āyurvedic system one can think about triple doshic functional integration which governs circulation and is felt in the deep pulse.

Feeble Circulation Pulse (Deep) under Ring Finger on the Right Side

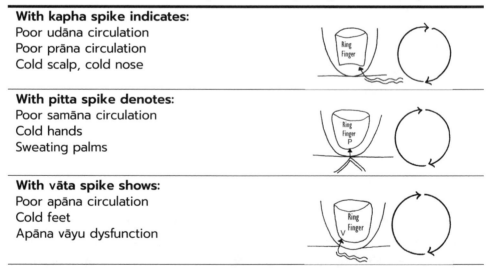

With kapha spike indicates:
Poor udāna circulation
Poor prāna circulation
Cold scalp, cold nose

With pitta spike denotes:
Poor samāna circulation
Cold hands
Sweating palms

With vāta spike shows:
Poor apāna circulation
Cold feet
Apāna vāyu dysfunction

Kapha affects circulation because the pulsations created in the heart are carried to the periphery, to the capillaries, due to the functional integration of the tridosha. Kapha doesn't allow the impulse to die. When kapha is not carrying sufficient impulse, the person will have poor circulation in the head. The scalp will be cold, the tip of the nose will be cold, sinuses will be congested and that person may faint.

On the other hand, due to excessive pitta rushing through the cerebral circulation, one can experience vertigo or dizziness and at the same moment, feel much heat in the scalp and the tip of the nose. Whenever we get a feeble circulation pulse under the ring finger, a kapha spike denotes poor circulation in the head. A feeble pulse with a pitta spike indicates poor circulation in the hands and sweating palms. A weak pulse with a vāta spike shows sluggish circulation in the lower extremities.

Small Intestine

Now we will switch our attention to the pulses on the subject's left side. The index finger at the superficial level corresponds to the small intestine. A spike at the kapha site, the proximal curvature, shows excess mucus in the small intestine, slow intestinal digestion or undigested fat in the small intestine which leads to fatty diarrhea called steatorrhea. The person with steatorrhea has difficulty digesting fat.

Feeble Small Intestine Pulse (Superficial) under Index Finger on the Left Side

With kapha spike indicates:
Excess mucus
Slow digestion
Undigested fat molecules
Fatty diarrhea

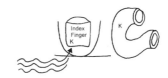

With pitta spike denotes:
Enteritis
Duodenal ulcer
Sprue syndrome
Chronic dysentery

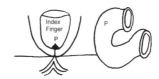

With vāta spike shows:
Hyperperistalsis
Partial obstruction
Thin intestinal wall
Malabsorption

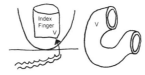

A spike at the central curvature of the index finger shows pitta in the intestines suggesting enteritis, duodenal ulcer, periumbilical burning sensation or sprue syndrome (malabsorption). The person has alternating diarrhea and constipation. Sprue syndrome is called chronic dysentery (*pitta grahani*).

A feeble small intestine pulse with a spike at the distal curvature (vāta) of the finger indicates hyperperistalsis, intestinal partial obstruction or intestinal colic. This condition may lead to a papery thin wall of the small intestine, causing chronic malabsorption syndrome (*gati yantra grahani*). In this condition the abdomen has a doughy feel indicating intestinal tuberculosis.

Grahani (Chronic Diarrhea). If the superficial pulse under the index finger on the left side of the subject becomes soft, feeble and infrequent, and the spike feels blunt at the pitta site, it denotes grahani, malabsorption syndrome in the small intestine.

Heart
The deep pulse at the seventh level under the index finger is the heart. It is composed of the heart muscle and the inner lining called the endocardium.

A kapha spike shows a slow heart, heart block, bundle branch block or myocardial hypertrophy with chronic or malignant hypertension called essential hypertension, which is common in older people. A kapha spike is a sign of high cholesterol and high triglycerides.

A strong pitta spike under the index finger denotes myocarditis, endocarditis or systemic high pitta in the heart. The heart is one of the seats of sādhaka pitta. When sādhaka pitta is high, a person becomes judgmental, critical, ambitious and competitive. A feeble heart pulse with a spike at pitta doesn't always mean endocarditis or myocarditis. It may be the pitta type of acute hypertension or a stressful condition due to a judgmental, critical, ambitious or competitive nature. Pitta hypertension is transient. A person becomes upset and, when he or she relaxes, the blood pressure becomes normal.

According to Āyurveda, one of the functions of sādhaka pitta in the heart is to transform feelings into emotions and maintain self-esteem. Depression can be vāta, pitta or kapha type. Kapha type of depression may be due to lack of sunlight. During the winter and on cloudy days one can feel depressed. Kapha type of depression may also be due to obesity, diabetes, hypertension, excess sleep or lethargy. Too much pitta in the heart may create depression. This type of depression may create thoughts of suicide and is associated with addiction to success or fear of failure. Pitta people tend to be perfectionists and, if a pitta person becomes aware that his or her judgment is wrong, depression may result. Vāta type of depression is associated with fear, anxiety, insecurity, and fear of the unknown, fear of tomorrow. Because of fear vāta individuals get depressed. When loss of control leads to depression, it is fear.

Vāta type of heart conditions includes tachycardia, atrial flutter with fibrillation, multiple extra systole, hypotension or alternating pulses. If vāta is in the heart, on inhalation the pulse becomes fast and on exhalation the pulse becomes slow. This condition is called sinus arrhythmia. Many times vāta in the heart creates pseudo-cardiac pain. A person may have palpitations, anxiety, insecurity or nervousness, but the reading of an electrocardiogram is absolutely normal. Palpitation means undue awareness of heart beat. Palpitation is normally present in exercise, excitation and anxiety. But pathologically, the person is aware of the heart beat even without exertion or exercise. That condition is called anxiety tachycardia, which is a prāna vāta disorder.

Feeble Heart Pulse (Deep) under the Index Finger on the Left Side

With kapha spike indicates:
Bradycardia
Bundle branch block
Myocardial hypertrophy
Malignant hypertension
High cholesterol

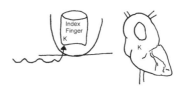

With pitta spike denotes:
Endocarditis
Ambition
Competitiveness
Anger
Hypertension

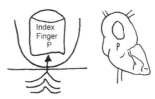

With vāta spike shows:
Depression
Fear
Anxiety
Tachycardia
Multiple extra systoles
Sinus arrhythmia

Some yogis stop their hearts through *prānāyāma* and awareness. The baby in the mother's womb listens to the heart sound and in deep meditation we listen to the music of the heart. A drum without fingers, a flute without lips and fingers, the heart sounds are felt as celestial, spiritual music. In meditation, by paying attention to the heart chakra, one will hear different sounds in the ear—the sound of the ocean, the sound of tabla and drum and ultimately leading to the sound of *Krishna*'s flute. When one hears the melody of a flute, all cows come together—cows mean senses—and they merge into Krishna, the higher consciousness within. Whenever one listens to the heart sound, there is a death of the ego and the ego doesn't like to die. Die to the ego, to power, prestige and position, then one will flow with the love, the inner sound, the primordial sound of his own prakruti. This sound is called "prakruti sound."

We are born with death. Death doesn't come from outside. As we grow, death also grows and the length of the death is exactly the length of the life. If we live 70 years, death lives with us 70 years. If we live 200 years, death lives with us 200 years. People fear death and that fear of death comes from attachment. We are attached to life and are afraid of seeing its end. At the deepest layer of life is neither birth nor death. In the heart there is a door and, if we meditate upon that door, we can jump into that layer of life which is beyond birth and death. That is meditation and meditation is the art of dying to the ego and to the body.

The heart is a most vital organ. When the heart stops, consciousness leaves the body in an ordinary person. But when a yogi stops his heart through yogic practice, his consciousness goes into the deeper layers of life beyond birth and death. That is called *samādhi* where there is no shadow of death. Samādhi means the art of going beyond birth and death. That is a state of balance.

The brain cells have a recording of death and birth. To take birth is very painful. If the child is asked how it feels to take birth, the child will say, "I was rejected. I was uprooted. I was thrown out of the Garden of Eden." The mother's womb is a Garden of Eden and the moment we become aware of our heartbeat, we are afraid.

Hrid Roga (Heart Disease in General)

The pulse at the site of the heart may show the following conditions:

1.) The pulse is feeble and beats like the swimming of a swan, indicating excess avalambaka kapha in the heart, myocardial hypertrophy.

2.) The pulse is feeble and beats like the hopping of a partridge, indicating congenital mitral valve prolapse.

3.) The pulse is frequent and moves like a collapsing plateau or mountain, indicating mitral incompetence.

4.) The pulse is irregularly irregular with cardiac arrhythmia and multiple extra systole, indicating atrial flutter with fibrillation.

5.) The kapha spike moves toward the pitta position which denotes kapha blocking pitta. The pulse feels like the mountain or crescendo pulse, indicating stenosis of the mitral valve with congestive cardiac failure.

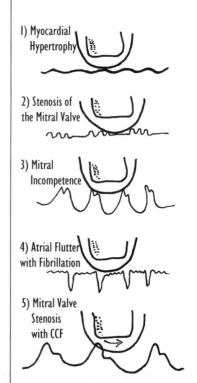

1) Myocardial Hypertrophy

2) Stenosis of the Mitral Valve

3) Mitral Incompetence

4) Atrial Flutter with Fibrillation

5) Mitral Valve Stenosis with CCF

Stomach

Under the middle finger the superficial pulse on the left hand of the subject is the stomach. A spike at the proximal curvature shows excess kledaka kapha in the stomach which will lead to low agni (manda agni), excessive mucous secretion, chronic indigestion, production of āma and low acidity. If this condition of hypochlorhydria, low acidity, remains for a long time, it can become pre-cancerous to the stomach. This condition should be treated by taking care of kapha through proper diet and herbal therapy.

Diagnosis can be confirmed by looking at the tongue. The tongue will show excess āma in the stomach area as shown in the diagram. There may be two spikes on the finger at the site of the stomach pulse, indicating excess pitta and excess kapha. A pitta spike denotes excess pitta and indicates over-secretion of hydrochloric acid. Pitta is increased by liquid quality, leading to low agni, which in turn causes acid indigestion, acute gastritis and peptic ulcer.

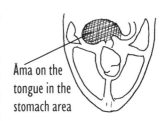

Āma on the tongue in the stomach area

Feeble Stomach Pulse (Superficial) under the Middle Finger on the Left Side

With kapha spike indicates:
Excess kledaka kapha in the stomach
Low agni (manda agni)
Chronic indigestion
Āma in the stomach
Hypochlorhydria (low hydrochloric acid)
Pre-diabetic condition

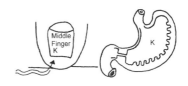

With pitta spike denotes:
Excess pāchaka pitta in the stomach
Hyperacidity
Strong appetite but poor digestion due to low agni and high pitta
Gastritis
Acid indigestion
Peptic ulcer

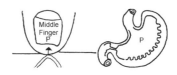

With vāta spike shows:
Hyperactivity in the stomach
Nervous stomach
Increased peristalsis
Vishama agni (irregular appetite)
Pyloric stenosis
Distended stomach
Gas in the fundus of the stomach
Narrow stomach

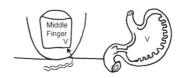

The presence of a vāta spike indicates imbalanced agni (vishama agni), irregular appetite and impaired digestion, gases in the fundus of the stomach and pyloric spasm. Even though pyloric stenosis is secondary to gastric ulcer, stenosis is due to vāta and a stomach deformity called hour glass constriction of the stomach. These are extreme vāta conditions as a complication to chronic pitta disorders. With esophageal problems the person can be asked where the food feels stuck. When the patient says the pain while swallowing is a sense of obstruction, if it is a man of 70, there is a possibility of cancer of the esophagus. But if an adult of 20 is complaining of tightness and a sense of obstruction of food, it may be due to anxiety, rapid eating or gas under the fundus. Hiatal hernia is a vāta disorder that should also be considered.

Mukha Pāka (Stomatitis, inflammation of oral mucous membrane).

When the stomach pulse shows a strong pitta spike that moves quickly with a snapping force, it indicates a stomach ulcer. As a complication, the person may get inflammation of the oral cavity or ulcers on the tongue. When there is food poisoning, the stomach pulse is feeble and shows high pitta, and the pulse partly disappears upon pressure. In this case, the patient may have symptoms such as nausea and vomiting.

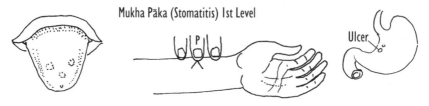

Mukha Pāka (Stomatitis) Ist Level

Spleen

The deep pulse at the seventh level under the middle finger on the left hand side of the person denotes the spleen (plīhā), and it can also be used to assess the pancreas. The spleen with a feeble spike at the kapha site indicates megaloblastic anemia, where the red blood cells are large in size but small in number. Or a kapha spike can indicate fluid in the abdominal cavity, which is called ascites. The spleen may be enlarged. *Yakrut* means liver and plīhā means spleen. Both are the root foundation of the hematopoietic system (rakta vaha srotas).

A pitta spike suggests splenitis and excess pitta in the spleen can create myeloid leukemia. In this condition a person bleeds—bleeding gums, rectum, the stomach and skin. Enlargement of the spleen can lead to anemia, a rañjaka pitta disorder. Red blood cells are broken and they become deformed as in sickle cell anemia or extreme hemolytic changes. The person then gets ascites with enlargement of the liver and spleen, which is called hepatosplenomegaly. When vāta is pushing pitta in the bone marrow (*majjā dhātu*), the ushna and tīkshna qualities of pitta disturb the red blood cells. Ask the subject if there has been a history of malaria or treatment with quinine. With pitta in the spleen, these possibilities are present. The spleen may be painful and tender in splenitis and the condition may develop into leukemia. What Āyurveda teaches makes great sense. Any dosha which is in the spleen may affect the immune system (ojas).

Feeble Spleen Pulse (Deep) under the Middle Finger on the Left Side

With kapha spike indicates:
Enlarged spleen
Megaloblastic anemia
Ascites
Swelling due to lymphatic obstruction

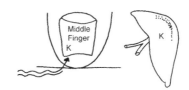

With pitta spike denotes:
Splenitis
Myeloid leukemia
Bleeding disorders
Enlarged tender spleen
Rañjaka pitta disorder
Hepatosplenomegaly
Ascites

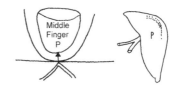

With vāta spike shows:
Aplastic anemia
Microcytic anemia
Splenic pain (vague)
Low immunity
Malaria

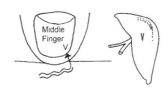

A vāta spike under the middle finger at the spleen site can lead to aplastic anemia, where the red blood cells are not properly formed; microcytic anemia, where the cells are smaller than normal size; splenic pain, extreme debility and low immunity. These conditions are very serious and not so common, but people frequently have low spleen energy. One shouldn't immediately jump to the conclusion of a serious condition but there is a possibility the person may go into anemia or blood borne disorders.

The production of red blood cells in the fetus takes place in the liver. The liver is the root of rakta vaha srotas. In the fetal body, the liver generates blood and the spleen creates white blood cells. Later on that function is slowly transferred to the bone marrow, which takes over the production of the red blood cells. The union of ossifying centers takes place at puberty. A radiologist, taking an x-ray of the joint, can tell the age of a person by observing the ossifying centers. At the age of puberty red blood cell formation is entirely transformed to the bone marrow via rañjaka pitta in the stomach.

The thymus gland (*adha jatru granthi*) produces specialized kapha molecules (white blood cells). These white blood cells are the policemen, the guards of the body, that catch bacteria and kill the viruses. The thymus gland in children is very active and large. It is the time of life when kapha is predominant and lymphocytes are associated with avalambaka kapha. In children the thymus gland produces more white blood cells to protect and maintain immunity. As the adult grows, the thymus gland becomes less active but is still important in maintaining immunity and supporting the body's normal function.

Madhumeha
(Glycosuria-Diabetes Insipidus)

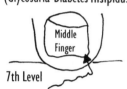

7th Level

Madhumeha (Glycosuria—Diabetes Insipidus). The deep pulse under the middle finger on the left side of the subject corresponds to both the spleen and pancreas and reveals the condition of the blood. If the pulse becomes thin like a hair and almost disappears with very little pressure, it indicates glycosuria. The spike is vāta in nature.

Plīhā Roga (Splenic Disorders). If the spleen pulse becomes feeble, thready and cold to the touch, and gives a vāta spike on the distal curvature, it indicates that the spleen is affected by vāta dosha. A vāta spike also shows low immunity, because the spleen plays an important role in the immune system. In cases of splenitis, the pulse will have a pitta spike in the middle of the curvature. A person having chronic fatigue syndrome may have pitta in the liver and spleen. In the case of splenomegaly, when the spleen is enlarged, there will be a kapha spike on the proximal curvature. Causes of enlarged spleen include infection, malaria and leukemia. Splenitis, a rañjaka pitta dysfunction, can also enlarge the spleen because of inflammation. The quality of the spike is very important in determining the nature of the disease.

Plīhā Roga (Splenic Disorders)
5th Level

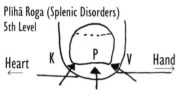

Heart

The immune system includes the digestive, endocrine and lymphatic systems. It also relies on proper functioning of the excretory system. Gently tapping the sternum stimulates the thymus gland, which in turn stimulates the immune mechanism. Immunity is also based upon positive thinking and functional balance between prāna, tejas and ojas. Negative thinking adversely affects prāna, tejas and ojas, the thymus gland, the spleen, the function of the lymphatic system and the entire immune system. With positive thinking, right attention and right intention, one can inject right awareness. Positive thinking strengthens the function of prāna, tejas and ojas and the thymus gland. The thymus gland is very close to the heart, which is the seat of emotions, and any negative emotion will first affect the thymus gland. During extreme stress and negative thinking, one's white blood cell count goes down.

Body, mind and spirit all need to be considered in holistic medicine. Modern doctors are learning ancient Āyurvedic concepts and body/mind medicine and are becoming more aware of spiritual aspects. Perhaps in the twenty-first century spirituality and medicine will go together. The spirit and mind cannot be separated from the body and the body/mind machine works as a unit. Āyurveda says that the body is not a mindless machine. The body is a dwelling of emotions, a house of spirit and the abode of consciousness. Body, mind and consciousness must be considered together.

Bladder

The last example of the superficial pulse on the left hand side of the subject, found under the ring finger, is the urinary bladder, or *mūtrāshaya*. The other name for bladder is *basti*. In pañchakarma the word basti is used to refer to a therapeutic enema. In ancient times the bladder of a horse or a buffalo was used to hold the liquid for an enema. The opening at the top of the bladder was tied to a bamboo tube, creating the ancient basti apparatus.

If the bladder pulse is feeble, try to locate the spike. A kapha spike with low bladder energy shows excess kapha in the bladder. Just give a kapha-soothing diet and the condition will be corrected. But if this condition remains, the person will get proteinuria (albuminuria), because kapha resembles protein molecules and will cause the patient to pass albumin in the urine. Another indication may be excess urination, polyuria, which is a sign of early diabetes. In cases of diabetes, which is a kapha disorder, kledaka kapha goes into the kidney and hence into the bladder. The urine will be cloudy, turbid and milky.

In pregnancy, because of the enlarged uterus which presses the bladder, a woman has frequent urination, which may be a kapha condition. A pregnant woman builds more kapha in her body in order to nourish the fetus. Kapha conditions include polyuria, diabetes, frequent urination, cloudy turbid urination and, in some cases, seminuria when a person passes semen in the urine. However, that semen doesn't go into the bladder; it comes out through the prostatic urethra.

A pitta spike indicates excess pitta in the bladder which may create repeated attacks of cystitis, inflammation of the bladder, burning urination, dark yellow color in the urine and sometimes blood in the urine. Hepatitis is a rañjaka pitta disorder in the liver, which creates excess secretion of bile salts, bile pigment and bilirubin. These secretions (rañjaka pitta) go into the bladder and pass out of the body through the urine. So excess pitta in the bladder can create bilirubinuria (bilirubin in the urine). That's why the urine is dark yellow, the color of turmeric. A B-complex vitamin supplement that is not utilized by the body also creates yellow-colored urine. If a person eats beets, the urine will be red. If the liver pulse is feeble and shows a pitta spike, there is a stagnation of rañjaka pitta in the liver. Hepatitis may not be active at present, but there may be a history of mononucleosis or hepatitis in the past. This rañjaka pitta is released into the bladder causing yellowish discoloration.

Feeble Bladder Pulse (Superficial) under Ring Finger on the Left Side

With kapha spike indicates:
Hyaline cast (mucus in the bladder)
Albuminuria (proteinuria)
Polyuria
Diabetes
Cloudy, turbid urination
Seminuria

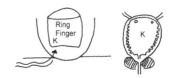

With pitta spike denotes:
Cystitis
Burning urination
Dark, yellow-colored urine
Hepatitis (bilirubinuria)
Acidic pH of urine
Hematuria (blood in the urine)

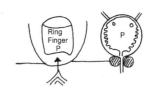

With vāta spike shows:
Scanty urination
Cold urine
Debilitated kidneys
Renal failure
Incontinence

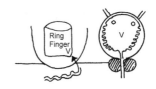

A vāta spike and low bladder energy may denote scanty urination, because urine is not properly filtered through the kidney. Even in the early morning such a person passes absolutely clear urine and the urine is foamy with bubbles. In addition, the urine is cold, as if one is passing cold water through the urethra. While passing urine, the person gets goose pimples, which is an early sign of debilitated kidney function leading to diabetes. In some conditions, urine is not formed at all in the kidneys, so excess vāta in the bladder may lead to anuria or suppression of urine. The bladder is totally empty, which in turn affects prāna and may lead to uremic coma.

Foam in the urine is due to a vāta dosha disorder. Anxiety and insecurity stimulate the bladder causing polyuria (excessive secretion of urine). Juvenile diabetes is a vāta disorder causing emaciation of the muscles. In this condition one gets a vāta spike under the ring finger.

Mūtrakrichra (Strangury). A vāta spike at the bladder pulse indicates retention of urine, because apāna vāyu doesn't open the sphincter muscle of the urethra. A pitta spike suggests excess pitta with acidic pH and that person may get cystitis or inflammatory conditions of the bladder. If a kapha spike is present, the person has albuminuria, diabetes or calcium phosphate stones. If the stone is an oxalate stone (pitta stone), it will cause bleeding and create a pitta spike on the pulse. Interstitial cystitis will show as both kapha and pitta spikes.

Mūtrakrichra (Strangury)
1st Level

Kidney

The deep pulse under the ring finger on the left hand side of the subject is the kidney pulse. If the kidney energy is low with a spike at the kapha site, kapha may drain the kidney energy, which will lead to albuminuria. Unabsorbed calcium molecules lodged in the kidney create crystalluria and these calcium crystals can lead to calcium stones. Other conditions caused by kapha are diabetes, hypertension, polycystic kidney, hydronephrosis and glycosuria. A person who consumes too much caffeine, sugar and milk may get excess kapha and a dull aching pain in the kidney. If a kapha pulse is felt in the kidney, one should shift to kapha-pacifying food.

Pitta in the kidney pulse shows excess pitta in the kidney, leading to nephritis or infection of the urinary tract, acute glomerulonephritis and hypertension. Pitta attracts oxalate crystals. Eating tomatoes, spinach and radishes, which are all rich in oxalic acid, may lead to the pitta type of oxalate stone. So people having kidney stones will have a kapha pulse, a pitta pulse or a kapha/pitta pulse, which means pitta is pushing kapha in the kidney. The result is calcium stones, oxalate stones or calcium-oxalate stones. The Bowman's capsule, which is a subtle mūtra vaha srotas, is located in the cortex of the kidney. Within the Bowman's capsule there is a network of capillaries called glomerulus. Acute glomerulonephritis, a high pitta condition in the kidney, will lead to hypertension, oxalate stones or fever, creating a burning pain in the renal angle.

Vāta in the kidney causes floating kidney, which means the kidneys are descended. Some people are born with kidneys that never grow to full size (juvenile small kidney), or one kidney is small and one kidney is normal. These people have vāta dosha in the kidney. Other conditions include oliguria, anuria, extreme fatigue, lower backache, phosphate crystals in the kidneys or phosphaturia, leading to calcium phosphate stones. Renal failure may result in uremic coma.

Feeble Kidney Pulse (Deep) under the Ring Finger on the Left Side

With kapha spike indicates:
Diabetes
Hypertension
Polycystic kidney
Hydronephrosis
Glycosuria
Calcium crystalluria

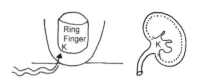

With pitta spike denotes:
Acute glomerulonephritis
Hypertension
Oxalate crystalluria
Burning pain in the kidney
Too much heat in the kidney

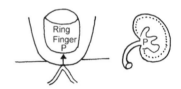

With vāta spike shows:
Renal failure
Congenital small kidney
Oliguria
Anuria
Extreme fatigue
Backache
Cold kidney
Floating kidney
Phosphaturia

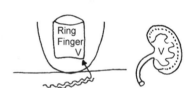

Shotha (Edema). If both feet are swollen with edema, the kidney pulse shows a kapha spike at the kapha site. The nature of the pulse is full, broad, wavy and slow and stops at times like a pillar. This condition indicates shotha, swelling on both feet. Due to accumulation of water under the skin, initially one may not be able to feel the pulse. But this pulse can be felt by repeated practice when water is displaced by the pressure of the finger.

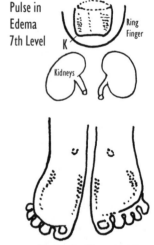

Shotha - Swelling in both Feet

INFLUENCE OF THE SEASONS ON THE PULSE

The rotation and movement of the earth are responsible for chronological time; both the days and seasons. The Sanskrit word for season is *rutu* and each rutu has specific qualities that can influence the bodily doshas. These qualitative seasonal variations can affect the qualities that are felt in the pulse, so one must take these into account when reading someone's pulse.

Summer is the season of pitta dosha, and it can cause high pitta in the system. This can influence the vikruti pulse, which will show a pitta spike. The same is true for fall, or autumn, which is a season of vāta dosha. The majority of clients will show a vāta spike in the vikruti pulse at this time of the year. Winter is the most healthy season, but it can lead to increased kapha and vāta. Hence many people get an extra kapha or vāta spike in the pulse in the wintertime. Finally, spring is a season when accumulated kapha begins to melt. Therefore, many clients show an extra kapha spike in this season.

THE BIOLOGICAL CLOCK AND THE PULSE: A SYMBOLIC REPRESENTATION

Time is a gradual movement. Each organ has a particular time of day when its functional activity is at a peak. One could think of this as the organs' biological clock, which moves with chronological time. The rising and setting of the sun determine chronological time, so although the sun actually rises and sets every day at a different time, for the convenience of understanding, we will assume the sun rises at 6:00 AM and examine the biological times for each organ.

The two hours after sunrise, which would be 6:00 to 8:00 AM, is lung time. A patient of bronchiectasis or mucous problems gets more pulmonary congestion at this time of day and it is also a good time to do prānāyāma. These two hours following sunrise relate to avalambaka kapha. From 8:00 to 10:00 is the time for *kloma*, the pancreas, an organ associated with kapha dosha, which regulates sugar and water metabolism. It also correlates to the spleen, another organ that is related to both kapha and pitta. At 10:00 AM, pitta time begins and the stomach and small intestine secrete pitta enzymes and stomach acid, which stimulates hunger. From 12:00 to 2:00 PM is heart time. The heart constantly circulates the blood and after a full meal, a person is more prone to a heart attack. From 2:00 to 4:00 PM is liver and gallbladder time, when a patient of hepatitis or coleocystitis is more likely to have a gallbladder attack. From 4:00 to 6:00 PM is the time of the ascending colon and kidneys. If kidney energy is low, a person may feel tired and want the boost from a cup of coffee to make them feel energetic during this time.

After sunset, the same pattern of organs repeats itself. Hence 6:00 to 8:00 PM is once again kapha and lungs time, when people have more congestion and an asthma patient may begin wheezing. Between 8:00 and 10:00 PM is pancreas and spleen time, and people who are hypoglycemic feel like munching before going to bed, because the pancreas becomes more active. Once again, 10:00 to 12:00 is stomach and small intestine time and pitta is active. At midnight, because acidity is very high in the stomach, an active peptic ulcer is more likely to create perforation. Then 12:00 to 2:00 AM is again heart time. Although the heart is resting, a person may have a heart attack during that time, due to the consumption of a late dinner. If a person has sex after a heavy meal, he could have a heart attack while making love. After having dinner at 6:00 o'clock, one can enjoy sex in the time frame of 9:00 to 10:00 in the evening. After 10 o'clock, one should not have sex but should go to sleep. However, people do not follow the laws of nature. They eat at 10 or 11 o'clock, go to bed at midnight, and then try to enjoy sex. It is disrespectful to the heart. Finally, from 2:00 to 4:00 AM is again liver and gallbladder time, which are related to rañjaka pitta, and 4:00 to 6:00 AM represents the descending colon and bladder.

One can take a person's pulse at any time, although as stated earlier, it is preferable to read it on an empty stomach. However, one should always take the time when the pulse is felt into consideration, noting the organ that is activated at that time. With this background, again choose a partner and feel the superficial and deep pulses. For every weak organ pulse, try to understand whether it is vāta, pitta or kapha that is affecting the organ and also check if it is a functionally active or inactive time of the day for that particular organ.

Biological Clock and the Pulse

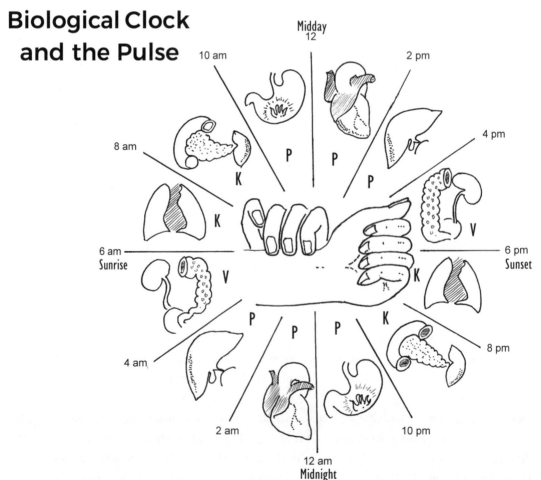

Table 6: Herbs for Treating Organ Disorders

Pulse Locations	1 Index Finger	2 Middle Finger	3 Ring Finger
1ST LEVEL	COLON	GALLBLADDER	PERICARDIUM
RIGHT HAND	Triphala Sat isabgol Senna Castor Oil Ajwan Hing	Ginger (fresh) Black pepper Piper longum Jatamāmsi Aloe vera juice Olive oil	Pushkarmūla Gulvel sattva Betel nut Ginger Cinnamon Nutmeg
7TH LEVEL	LUNGS	LIVER	CIRCULATION
RIGHT HAND	Piper longum Punarnava Abhrak bhasma Kantakāri Tulsi (Holy basil, sweet basil) Yashthi madhu	Kutki Shankha pushpi Neem Aloe vera gel Manjishthā Tikta Shilājit	Trikatu Cinnamon Cardamom Clove Turmeric Cayenne pepper Manjishthā Red sandalwood
	1 Index Finger	2 Middle Finger	3 Ring Finger
1ST LEVEL	SMALL INTESTINE	STOMACH	BLADDER
LEFT HAND	Chitrak Gulwel sattva Danti Kāma dudha Cumin Pippalī Saffron Hing	Shatāvarī Yashthi madhu Shankha bhasma Ajwan Amalaki Mustard Cumin Ginger Saffron	Punarnava Amalaki Cumin Gokshura Coriander Fennel Chandan (white) Coconut
7TH LEVEL	HEART	SPLEEN	KIDNEYS
LEFT HAND	Arjuna Cinnamon Gudūchī Amalaki Tagara Nutmeg Passion flower Hawthorn berry Manuka Pomegranate	Manjishthā Saffron Turmeric Shilājit Echinacea Osha Mahāsudarshana	Punarnava Gokshura Shilājit Cilantro Mūtrala Ashvagandha Vidhari

4

SUBTYPES OF THE DOSHAS
Through the Pulse
Level Three

Vāta, pitta and kapha govern different aspects of physiology, as we have already discussed. In addition, each dosha has five functional subtypes. Vāta is composed of prāna, udāna, samāna, vyāna and apāna. Pitta is subdivided into pāchaka, rañjaka, *ālochaka*, sādhaka and *bhrājaka*. Kapha consists of kledaka, avalambaka, bodhaka, tarpaka and shleshaka. Each of these subtypes represents a particular aspect of physiology.

The Āyurvedic theory of five elements is a basic concept about the creation of the universe and man. This concept continues even into the subtypes of the doshas. The five subtypes of each dosha contain all five elements, but one particular element is most prominent for each. For example, out of the vāta subtypes, ether is most prominent for prāna, air is for udāna, fire for samāna, water for vyāna, and earth element for apāna. The same holds true for the five subtypes of pitta and kapha.

Every dosha has a gati, which means movement, and each of the subtypes has its own particular gati. Again, to use vāta as an example, upward movement is udāna, downward movement is apāna, inward is prāna, linear is samāna, and circulatory movement is vyāna. If the dosha is moving in a circular manner, it is vyāna. To understand the disease process and the vector of samprāpti (pathogenesis), a knowledge of the subtypes is important.

The subtypes of each dosha are significant as indicators of qualitative or pre-pathological changes, as opposed to the quantitative changes seen in vikruti that lead to pathology. These subtypes are read on the third level of the radial pulse. To do this, first place the fingers on the first level, where vikruti is felt. Then pass through the second level and, with a bit more pressure, become aware of the third level of the pulse. The index finger still shows vāta, the middle finger pitta, and the ring finger is kapha. In addition, each fingertip has five sites where a spike can be felt—one for each subdosha.

A spike at one of these five positions indicates an involvement of that particular doshic subtype. To use the vāta subtypes as an example, a spike at the distal curvature of the index finger is prāna, while a little closer to the middle curvature is udāna. Then on the other side of the curvature is samāna and at the extreme end is apāna. Vyāna is felt in the middle, as shown in the diagram.

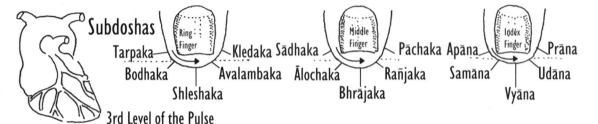

The more closely we observe, the more we understand. Suppose a person has a problem with a number of vāta symptoms. Which subtype or subtypes of vāta dosha are primarily involved? The third level pulse felt by the index finger will reveal whether it is prāna, udāna, samāna, apāna or vyāna, because the subtype/s out of balance will create a spike. The finger is a sensitive electrode when it is placed on the pulse to find the location of any spike. The quality of the pulse is also important, but at the early stage of learning, just be aware of the position of the spike and learn which subtype is taking part in the disease process (samprāpti).

The same principle is applied to the middle finger for detecting disorders of the subtypes of pitta dosha, and the ring finger for disorders of the kapha subtypes, as shown in the illustration. Note that the arrow in the diagram shows the direction of blood flow. There is some difference in opinion about the location of sādhaka and ālochaka pitta, but this is the order I have learned from my experience. Bhrājaka pitta is located on the central curvature and moves across the proximal curvature of the finger.

There is a relationship between the serial order of the subtypes, as can be illustrated using kapha dosha subtypes on the ring finger. Kledaka kapha is located at the extreme distal curvature, next is avalambaka and then bodhaka and tarpaka. Finally, shleshaka is located on the central curvature. Kledaka nourishes avalambaka, while avalambaka supports bodhaka, which enlivens tarpaka. More simply, kledaka nourishes avalambaka, which nourishes all kapha systems. Again, some would switch tarpaka and bodhaka, but these are the locations that I learnt from my mentor.

Now feel your own pulse and see which subtype of each dosha is active at present. If you feel a strong spike, it indicates that the dosha subtype is hyperactive (*dosha vruddhi*). Any feeble spike means that the subtype is underactive (dosha kshaya). The subtypes can indicate physiology as well as pathology, so how can one detect whether it is physiological activity or pathological activity? One important thing is that a general movement from the heart toward the periphery of the body is a sign of normal physiological activity. For instance, when vyāna vāyu propels the circulation from the heart to the periphery, normal physiological activity is present. Whereas if vyāna moves retrograde, from the periphery back to the heart, it denotes a pathological condition such as congestion or altered cardiac function. This applies to any subtype. During ancient times, there were no x-rays or other modern equipment, so the physicians of that time read the pulse and tried to diagnose the problem by understanding the quality, nature and direction of the spike.

If the third level of the pulse is felt in the morning, afternoon and evening, and if one subtype of a dosha is persistently moving in a retrograde direction, consider the possibility that there is some kind of abnormality. A retrograde flow can result in severe tissue damage and it may lead to complications.

Go step by step. Using the chart of the finger positions, feel each subtype that has a spike and note down which subtype of the dosha is out of balance.

VĀTA DOSHA SUBTYPES

A dysfunction in a doshic subtype can manifest in specific ways. Considering first the subtypes of vāta, a spike under the vāta finger at the prāna site can denote a migraine type of headache, ringing in the ears, dizziness or some mental dysfunction such as chattering of the brain, thinking too much, insomnia, interrupted sleep or excessive dreaming. Swallowing is a function of prāna, so dysphasia (difficulty in swallowing), hurried eating and hiccoughs are other dysfunctional disorders of prāna, along with loss of sensory and motor responses.

Udāna governs speech, recollection, belching and hiccoughing, because udāna moves upward. Udāna vāyu is also responsible for effort, energy and color complexion as well as memory retention. Prāna gives light to the memory, but it is udāna that makes memory function according to time and space. Udāna works at the throat chakra and it enables communication and the expression of thoughts, feelings and emotions.

Udāna and prāna pulses can be confusing to feel, because they are so close together on the finger. If it is difficult to determine their exact location, just write down both prāna and udāna and then later, as you observe more closely, it will become clear which one is correct. If it is prāna, other symptoms connected to the respiratory or nervous

Subtypes of Vāta Dosha

Apāna — Prāna
Samāna — Udāna
Vyāna

system will manifest. If it is udāna that is involved, there may be hiccoughs, breathlessness, poor memory or fatigue.

If samāna is affected, there may be a digestive disorder or mal-absorption syndrome, because digestion, absorption, assimilation and intestinal peristalsis are all governed by samāna. Similarly, apāna is related to elimination and vyāna to circulation. Apāna normally stays in the colon and pelvic cavity, and it governs the functions of the bladder, rectum, menstruation, ovulation and ejaculation. Whenever apāna vāyu is affected, ask the person about these functions. Is elimination functioning properly? Is menstruation painful? Does the person have low backache, sciatica, premature ejaculation, painful ovulation or premenstrual syndrome?

Finally, a spike at the site of vyāna vāyu is connected to a disorder of circulation, blood pressure, or the joints, especially the reflexes. It may be responsible for tremors, tics and spasms, although nervous disorders in general are connected to prāna.

PITTA DOSHA SUBTYPES

Within the subtypes of pitta, pāchaka governs digestion, absorption and assimilation of food. If a pāchaka pitta spike is persistent at the third level, there is some kind of disease process going on and digestion may be affected.

Rañjaka pitta is associated with the liver and spleen and a feeble spike at this site may indicate a weak liver, jaundice, hepatitis, gallstones, mononucleosis or chronic fatigue syndrome. It is involved in the creation of red blood cells (RBC), so a dysfunction of rañjaka may cause anemia. In the stomach, rañjaka pitta can be compared to the gastric intrinsic factor, which is necessary for erythrogenesis, the formation of red blood cells. A rañjaka pitta disorder may also indicate a spleen or stomach dysfunction, high cholesterol or high triglycerides.

Ālochaka pitta is present in the eyes—retina, lens, color vision, optical perception and visual acuity. Ālochaka dysfunction may manifest as conjunctivitis, blepharitis, glaucoma, burning sensations in the eyes, 'floaters' and increased intraocular pressure. In cases of cataracts, pitta pushes kapha and the kapha molecules lodge in the lens and make it smoky, cloudy and opaque.

Sādhaka pitta is present in the brain and heart. It is responsible for understanding, knowledge, comprehension, appreciation, self-esteem, confidence, courage and the capacity to express thoughts and feelings. In the heart, it processes feelings into emotions. When sādhaka pitta is dysfunctional, a person may make the wrong conclusions and have confusion, delusions, or hallucinations. Sādhaka pitta synthesizes words into knowledge and processes information into comprehension. It is responsible for concentration, attention and maintaining perception. When sādhaka pitta is adversely affected, there is poor concentration, lack of attention and unclear perception. Sādhaka digests and transforms information into knowledge. When knowledge is not there, then memory is not there, although memory is not directly connected to sādhaka pitta; it is the function of udāna vāyu.

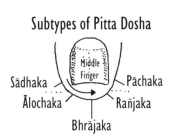

Subtypes of Pitta Dosha

Bhrājaka pitta is present under the skin and maintains the normal color of pigmentation cells. It processes every tactile sensation of touch, pain and temperature. This perception is called stereognosis—stereo means three-dimensional and gnosis means knowledge. Because of touch perception, a blind man recognizes common objects, such as a key, coins or matchbox. A blind person can even read through touch. The skin has a deep understanding of touch and a person knows if he or she is being touched with love or sexuality, or perhaps anger, hate or fear. These subtle understandings of the meaning of touch are the functions of bhrājaka pitta. If someone touches with great love, bhrājaka pitta processes that touch into healing love.

When insufficient light falls on the skin of the forehead, a person can become depressed. Depression is uncommonly common in the winter, because of insufficient light being received by bhrājaka pitta. If exposed to full spectrum light, bhrājaka pitta secretes serotonin via sādhaka pitta, which is necessary to avoid depression. Eczema, dermatitis, psoriasis, acne, hives, rash, urticaria and erysipelas are other common bhrājaka pitta disorders. A dysfunction of bhrājaka pitta is also involved in skin cancer and one way to prevent this is by the application of neem oil on the skin. Neem oil acts as a partial sun blocker.

Note that rañjaka pitta maintains the color of bhrājaka pitta, which maintains the color of the skin. In anemia the skin becomes pale, because rañjaka pitta doesn't produce enough red blood cells to color bhrājaka. If there is excess rañjaka pitta, the person may get polycythemia and red, flushed skin. There is functional integrity between rañjaka pitta and bhrājaka pitta and also between ālochaka and rañjaka. Ālochaka pitta and rañjaka pitta work together to maintain the color of the iris.

KAPHA DOSHA SUBTYPES

Moving now to the kapha subtypes, kledaka kapha is present in the stomach and gastrointestinal tract as well as rasa dhātu, and it aids in the digestion, absorption and assimilation of foodstuff. Dysfunctional kledaka kapha affects digestion in the stomach, duodenum and jejunum. If a kledaka kapha spike is persistently detected, one should think about diabetes as a possible pathological condition.

Avalambaka kapha is present in the lungs, pleura, pericardium, bronchi, bronchioles and alveoli. Avalambaka kapha enters the heart, circulates throughout the body and nourishes all kapha systems. A spike at avalambaka kapha indicates a possibility of bronchial congestion, pleural effusion, pneumonia, bronchitis or other lung conditions. It may also suggest a pericardial condition. A dysfunction of avalambaka kapha may cause pain in the mid-back. The thoracic vertebrae from T-4 through T-12 are connected to the mediastinum and mid-back tightness. Emotional aspects of avalambaka kapha manifest as unresolved, deep-seated grief and sadness in the lungs. A history of smoking or inhaling drugs like cocaine may also affect avalambaka.

Bodhaka kapha is associated with the mouth, tongue, gums and teeth. It is present in the saliva, where it governs the digestion of carbohydrates and assists in general digestion via kledaka kapha. If bodhaka kapha is involved, the person may have receding gums, gum abscesses or dental cavities. Taste is related to rasa dhātu and bodhaka kapha is directly connected to rasa. Bodhaka kapha perceives the different tastes—sweet, sour, salty, bitter, pungent, astringent—and its dysfunction can create a perverted taste in the mouth. The saliva may taste salty even though no salt is eaten, or the mouth may have a bitter taste without the consumption of a bitter substance. All six tastes must be present equally for balance. If rasa lacks sufficient sweet or sour taste, for example, then there is a craving for sweet or sour. The patient of diabetes has a craving for sweet and may experience a sweet taste in the mouth. Bodhaka kapha dysfunction can be expressed through the pulse in people who are diabetic or hypersensitive to sugar and carbohydrates.

Tarpaka kapha is associated with the brain meninges and the white matter. The functional element of the gray matter is sādhaka pitta and the white matter is tarpaka kapha. Tarpaka is also present in the sinuses and the middle ear and is the material from which a neuron is formed. *Tarpanam* means nourishing, including the senses. All sensory perceptions—auditory, tactile, optical, gustatory, and olfactory—are carried to tarpaka kapha by prāna vāyu. The job of tarpaka kapha is to nourish every sensory perception and to store those perceptions as concrete experience. Every experience that has been processed by sādhaka pitta is crystallized and recorded on the sensitive film of tarpaka kapha. Functionally, tarpaka is connected to the astral body. All past life memories, experiences and knowledge are stored within the matrix of tarpaka kapha. Neurotransmitters are included in sādhaka pitta and these neurotransmitters are responsible for the synthesis and processing of acetylcholine into serotonin and melatonin. While this transformation into consciousness, alertness, happiness and knowledge is the function of sādhaka pitta, all these functions take place on the screen of tarpaka kapha. When watching a movie, one needs light. That light is sādhaka pitta and the projecting factor is prāna, but the movie screen is tarpaka kapha. Therefore, there is a functional integration between prāna vāyu, the projector, tarpaka kapha, the screen, and sādhaka pitta, the light. Without that screen, no movie of life is possible.

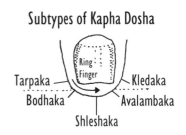

Subtypes of Kapha Dosha

Paralysis is classified into vāta, pitta and kapha types and tarpaka kapha is involved in stroke paralysis. A dysfunction of tarpaka kapha can create increased intra-cranial pressure, dizziness, sinus congestion and sensory tiredness. These dysfunctions can aggravate prāna, which pushes aside tarpaka kapha and creates spaciness and dizziness. In order to protect the body, tarpaka kapha tries to control prāna. Prāna is often more powerful and mental fatigue is connected to such a disorder of prāna vāta and tarpaka kapha.

The last doshic subtype is shleshaka kapha, which is present in all the joints and governs lubrication. A spike under the ring finger at the shleshaka kapha site may suggest tightness and stiffness of the joints, cracking and popping of the joints, or arthritis.

In this way, the third level pulse of each subtype of the doshas can reveal various physio-pathological changes that take place in the body. One must practice reading each of these fifteen subtypes' pulses with great awareness and find the ones that have a spike, indicating that the particular subdosha is working under stress.

5

DHĀTUS THROUGH THE PULSE
The Examination of Biological Tissues
Level Five

The fifth level of the pulse represents the dhātus or biological tissues—rasa, plasma; rakta, blood tissue; *māmsa*, muscle tissue; *meda*, fat and adipose tissue; asthi, bone; majjā, bone marrow and nerve tissue; *shukra*, male reproductive tissue and *ārtava*, female reproductive tissue.

Prakruti, which is felt at the deepest level of the pulse, is the most consistent of the pulses. The dhātu or tissues pulse also reflects a deep layer of physiology. Longstanding imbalances due to āma and doshic influences show up in this layer of pulse, if the dhātu agni is debilitated. The condition of dhātu agni relates to the quantitative and qualitative production of that tissue. For example, high dhātu agni causes depletion of the tissue, while weak dhātu agni causes accumulation of unprocessed raw tissue. A spike under the palpating finger at the dhātu level shows a tissue agni that is working under stress.

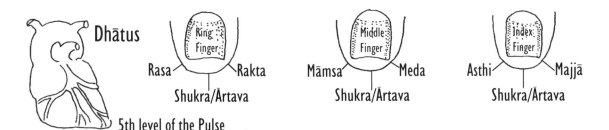

Dhātus

Ring Finger

Rasa — Rakta

Shukra/Ārtava

Middle Finger

Māmsa — Meda

Shukra/Ārtava

Index Finger

Asthi — Majjā

Shukra/Ārtava

5th level of the Pulse

First, we will try to find the fifth level. Step by step, go from the skin down to the fifth level, or by first going to the seventh level and then passing up through the sixth level—the level of manas prakruti, which we have not yet discussed—and releasing slowly to feel the fifth. Normally, a healthy dhātu doesn't show any spike. But if a dhātu is weak and is affected by vāta, pitta or kapha, a spike will be present.

Find the location of each dhātu (refer to the diagram) and feel if there is any spike, to determine if that particular dhātu is working under stress or if it is weak. Any of the doshas can move through the dhātus, so the quality of the spike is very

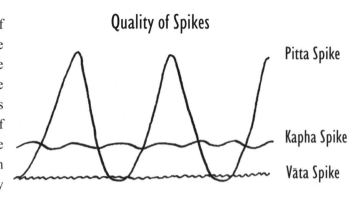

Quality of Spikes

Pitta Spike

Kapha Spike

Vāta Spike

important. A delicate, thready, feeble spike is vāta. If it is sharp and uplifting, it indicates pitta. If it is dull and moderate, it is kapha. For example, if there is a vāta spike under the site of rasa, this means vāta is weakening rasa dhātu. Similarly, a kapha spike at the meda site indicates kapha in *meda dhātu*.

If you feel a spike along the central part of the tip of any of the three fingers, there is involvement of a dosha affecting shukra or ārtava. If this spike is under the ring finger, there may be excess kapha in the shukra or ārtava. If this spike is beneath the middle finger, there is excess pitta; and a spike at the central curvature of the index finger indicates excess vāta in shukra or ārtava dhātu. Healthy dhātus don't allow the doshas to "escape" through the pulse. But if the dhātu is weak, the doshas are present in the pulse and can be felt.

KALĀ

In order to deepen our understanding, we must consider the concept of *kalā*. A kalā is a membranous structure that is a protective barrier between two tissues. It maintains the nutrition, transformation and maturation of a dhātu and it contains the agni of that particular tissue as well as its prāna, tejas and ojas. If the dhātu agni within a kalā undergoes an increased or decreased condition, it may cause atrophy or hypertrophy of that particular dhātu. If the agni of the kalā is low, there is undue accumulation of raw dhātu. If *kalā agni* is high, the dhātu will be emaciated.

Each of the dhātus has its own kalā. For instance, rasa dhātu (plasma) and rakta dhātu (red blood cells), as well as all the other tissues, are separated by a sheath. In this case, it is called *rakta dhārā kalā*. Within that kalā is the respective dhātu agni, which maintains the unique metabolism of the dhātu. So in rakta dhārā kalā, there is *rakta agni*. Similarly, between meda and asthi tissues is *asthi dhārā kalā* and it contains *asthi agni*.

Each dhātu follows a similar pattern of transformation. The immature tissue is processed into mature tissue, along with the formation of by-products and *malas* (wastes), plus the production of the immature form of the following tissue. For example, unprocessed rasa dhātu is transformed into four main substances: processed rasa, immature rakta, the by-products of rasa—*stanya* (lactation) and *rajah* (menstruation)—and kapha, which is the *dhātu mala*.

When food is eaten, *āhāra rasa* (chyle), the food precursor for cellular nourishment, is produced within six to eight hours. Within 24 hours, immature rasa dhātu is created from āhāra rasa. The time required for *rasa dhārā kalā* to transform āhāra rasa into mature rasa dhātu is five days. Rakta dhārā kalā needs 10 days to produce mature rakta dhātu and fully processed māmsa dhātu requires 15 days. Likewise, it takes an additional five days for each dhātu, up to 35 days (just over one month) for shukra or ārtava dhātu to receive the full benefit of nutrition from the food. Note that certain foods can nourish the immature form of a tissue within a short period of time. For example, milk is the highly superfine essence of the rasa dhātu of the cow and it is transformed into shukra within 24 hours. Hence, an Āyurvedic sūtra says "Milk nourishes shukra on the same day."

Āyurveda says *shukra dhārā kalā*, the kalā which nourishes shukra dhātu, the male reproductive tissue, and *ārtava dhātu kalā* in the female, are present all over the body. When one touches someone else with feelings of sex, it stimulates the agni of that shukra or ārtava kalā and activates sperm or ova. The entire body is covered by shukra or ārtava dhārā kalā, which produces ojas. Too much sex depletes ojas, which can then diminish the body's immune mechanism.

The Sanskrit word srotas or srotāmsi (plural) means channel. Every dhātu also has its corresponding channel and the root of that srotas is present in the kalā. Kalā is not an imagined, intellectual, poetic concept, but is an actual membranous structure. Each dhātu has its own intelligence, which is present within that membrane. The nucleus has a membrane, each gene has a membrane, and even each individual cell has a membrane.

The membranous structure of the genes and RNA/DNA molecules have their subtle kalās in which are carried the memories of our ancestors' illnesses.

Every organ has a mucous lining that maintains the normal functioning of that particular organ. This lining is also called kalā. *Āshaya* means vessel and every āshaya has a kalā. The stomach is a vessel of undigested food, called *āmāshaya*. It has a gastric mucous membrane called *shleshma dhārā kalā*. *Shleshma* means kapha. The small intestine has an intestinal mucous membrane called *pitta dhārā kalā*. The colon has a mucous membrane called *purisha dhārā kalā*. These three mucous membranes are protective coverings of the gastrointestinal tract.

When hot food is eaten—for example, hot cayenne pepper or chili—it stimulates the production of hydrochloric acid and dissolves the kalā of the stomach. This stimulates more production of kledaka kapha and within three to six hours, a new stomach mucous membrane lining, called shleshma dhārā kalā, is formed. The colon mucous membrane functionally corresponds to the periosteum. It is this purisha dhārā kalā which nourishes the periosteum, because the colon is the organ that absorbs minerals such as calcium, magnesium and zinc.

The root of all disease is weak agni, which leads to the formation of āma. There are many causes for this. For example, whenever incompatible foods are ingested, *jathara agni* will be directly affected and āma or toxins will be created from those poorly digested foods. Hyperactive agni also affects the digestive process through over-combustion, resulting in emaciation and lowered immunity.

The malfunction of any kalā creates āma in the related organ or dhātu. The main center of digestion and the most important agni is the gastric fire, jāthara agni, which is present in the stomach or āmāshaya. If someone has weak jāthara agni, it will result in āma formation in the GI tract. The kalā in the gastrointestinal tract maintains the functions of jāthara agni, while the functional aspects of dhātu agni are maintained by the *dhātu kalā*. However, there is functional integ-

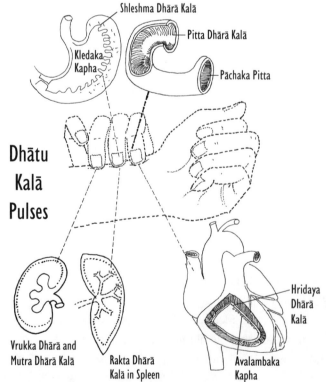

Dhātu Kalā Pulses

Shleshma Dhārā Kalā

Pitta Dhārā Kalā

Kledaka Kapha

Pāchaka Pitta

Hridaya Dhārā Kalā

Vrukka Dhārā and Mutra Dhārā Kalā

Rakta Dhārā Kalā in Spleen

Avalambaka Kapha

rity between the kalā in the GI tract and the kalā in the dhātus. Sometimes an individual may have strong jāthara agni but weak dhātu agni, and this condition can directly create āma in the dhātu. On the other hand, if jāthara agni is low and āma is produced, that āma can affect the dhātu agni and go into the dhātus. Any āma in the tissues is created by the malfunction of the dhātu kalā. For example, āma is created by the gastric mucous membrane when it is not properly secreting digestive enzymes and kledaka kapha.

Āma in the GI tract is not always created in the stomach. It can be produced in the colon because of constipation, or in an individual dhātu because of low dhātu agni or an infection. Āma can also form in the liver or gallbladder because of repressed emotions, such as anxiety, insecurity, nervousness, fear or anger. This is called mental āma, which is stored in the dhātus or organs.

Āyurvedic pharmacology discusses how certain herbs have specific actions on a particular dhātu agni or kalā. For example, ginger stimulates rasa dhārā kalā, manjishthā works on rakta dhārā kalā, ashvagandha activates *māmsa dhārā kalā*, kutki acts on *meda dhārā kalā*, guggulu on asthi dhārā kalā, brahmi on *majjā dhārā kalā*, atma gupta on shukra dhārā kalā and shatāvarī on ārtava dhārā kalā. There is a logical order in Āyurvedic anatomy, physiology and disease management, including Āyurvedic herbology.

DISORDERS OF THE DHĀTUS

Specific disorders of the dhātus may be present if a spike is found at the fifth level and we will now turn our attention to how these imbalances manifest in each of the tissues.

Rasa

If a vāta spike is felt at the rasa dhātu site, the person may have dehydration, dry skin, or poor circulation and cold skin. There is a possibility of blackish or brownish discoloration of the skin and the skin may become cracked and rough.

A pitta spike at the rasa site indicates that excess pitta is flowing through rasa dhātu leading to pyrexia (fever), hot flashes, acne, rash or eczema.

A kapha spike at the rasa dhātu site indicates the possibility of dermoid cysts, or the skin may become thick and even sclerodermic. Kapha in rasa dhātu also causes lymphatic congestion and kapha types of allergies, such as colds or sneezing. Don't jump directly to the conclusion of a serious condition. First rule out common conditions, such as a cold, congestion or cough.

Rakta

The second dhātu is rakta. A vāta spike at the rakta site shows a mild case of anemia. Also look for an abnormal pulsation in the external jugular vein. Vāta in rakta dhātu can create low blood pressure; the person may feel dizzy or have vertigo. There may also be cardiac arrhythmia. A vāta spike may also denote the condition of vāta rakta, which is gout.

A pitta spike at the rakta dhātu site may indicate bleeding disorders, such as bleeding gums, bleeding hemorrhoids, or bleeding in the gastrointestinal tract which makes the stool tarry black. Pitta in rakta can be related to hives, rashes and urticaria. The person may easily bruise. This condition of excess pitta may lead to sickle cell anemia, because high pitta burns the red blood cells and distorts the shape of the cells.

A kapha spike in rakta dhātu indicates high cholesterol, high triglycerides or hypertension. Blood sugar may be high. Kapha is sweet and kapha in rakta may show hyperglycemia or an inclination toward diabetes. All these disorders are not necessarily present, but there may be a predisposition or family history of these conditions, which can be detected through the pulse. The pulse might indicate some abnormality, but if the person has symptoms, it may be genetic. Taking the family medical history of the person will help to clarify this information.

Māmsa

A vāta spike at the *māmsa dhātu* site shows muscle tics, spasms, weakness, fatigue or twitching as well as improper coordination. Another condition that may be present is muscle atrophy, because vāta can create emaciation of the muscle.

A pitta spike at the māmsa site indicates myositis, bursitis and tendonitis. Long-standing pitta in māmsa dhātu may create muscular rheumatism, which is a general inflammatory condition creating a rheumatic type of pain. This condition indicates that sometime in the future the person may develop a rheumatic disorder or fibromyalgia. Other manifestations are multiple boils and hemorrhoids. Hemorrhoids can arise from the musculature of the blood vessel because of aggravated pitta. (Hemorrhoids can also be either vāta- or kapha-type.) The muscular layer of the blood vessel becomes irritated and inflamed, creating the piles (or hemorrhoids). Uvulitis creates a cough and irritation of the throat, which is also pitta in māmsa dhātu. In this condition, the uvula becomes inflamed and the irritation causes the uvula to lengthen, creating a blockage to the respiratory passage, which can lead to snoring.

A kapha spike at the māmsa dhātu position may indicate dermoid cysts or benign tumors, muscle tumors called myomas, and muscular hypertrophy, which means increased size of the muscle. Longstanding, lingering vāta in the muscles can create atrophy, whereas kapha creates hypertrophy. Growth is different from hypertrophy. When there is growth, the cells increase in number. In hypertrophy, the cells increase in size, resulting in one muscle or a group of muscles becoming unduly large. This observation can be equally true of skeletal or smooth muscles, because all muscle tissue comes under māmsa dhātu.

Meda

A vāta spike at the meda site indicates emaciation. Meda dhātu nourishes the synovia, so there will be lack of lubrication. Vāta in meda dhātu will eventually create dislocation of the joints, because of the drying of the synovial fluid and weakening of the ligaments.

A pitta spike at the meda dhātu location may indicate an inflammatory condition of the kidneys, adrenals or other organs related to meda. All round organs accumulate fat and, when there is excess pitta in meda dhātu, the person may develop fatty degenerative changes in the liver. Pitta in meda dhātu also creates acidic sweat and the person may get boils and abscesses.

A kapha spike at the meda dhātu site may indicate multiple lipomas, fibromas, fibrocystic breasts, renal calculi, gallstones and sebaceous cysts. Sebaceous cysts are located close to the midline of the body. Urine carries *kleda* (the liquid component of kapha) from meda dhātu. If there is excess pitta in meda dhātu, the kleda becomes acidic and creates nephritis. Due to nephritis a person gets hypertension. Nephritis begins with pitta but ends with kapha. Albuminuria will also be common if kapha is in meda dhātu.

Asthi

A vāta spike at the site of asthi dhātu may indicate cracking and popping of the joints, osteoporosis, and degenerative arthritis. The hair and nails may become brittle and cracked and the person may start losing hair, owing to brittleness. However, in this condition the hair can grow normally again once vāta calms down.

A pitta spike at the asthi site may indicate periostitis and severe loss of hair. Pubic and axillary hair will be lost when shukra or ārtava dhātu is affected, but this will affect hair on the head and can lead to baldness. The person may get repeated fungal infection of the nails or tooth abscesses.

A kapha spike at the asthi dhātu site may indicate osteoma, swollen joints with effusion and Koch's knee, which is tuberculosis of the knee joint. Kapha in asthi dhātu may also lead to deformities of the bones and nails.

Majjā

A vāta spike at the majjā dhātu site may indicate neurological symptoms such as tingling, numbness and loss of sensation. Sensory perception of touch, pain and temperature may be diminished. In its mild form, when vāta goes into the majjā the person may have insomnia, hyperactivity and raging thoughts. It can create strabismus (crossed eyes) and ptosis. Vāta in majjā dhātu can also affect māmsa and disturb the coordination and tone of the muscles.

Muscle tone is maintained by the integrity between tarpaka and shleshaka kapha, and prāna and vyāna vāyu. If this functional integration is disturbed, the person may develop either hypertonia (rigidity) or hypotonia (flaccidity). When tarpaka is involved, an upper motor neuron lesion leads to increased rigidity. Reflexes will be exaggerated (hypertonia) owing to the tarpaka kapha disorder. Hence by disturbing tarpaka kapha, vāta in majjā may lead to Parkinson's disease, epileptic fits, epilepsy and convulsions. In a shleshaka kapha disorder, which involves a lower motor neuron lesion, reflexes will be abolished. When vāta affects shleshaka in majjā dhātu, it will lead to loss of tone (hypotonia). The lower motor neurons contain shleshaka kapha within the intercellular spaces of majjā dhātu as well as in the joints. A lower motor neuron type of paralysis creates rapid muscle wasting and changes such as ulceration of the tissues. These are serious conditions and stroke paralysis is a classical example. Depending upon whether the lesion affects the upper or lower motor neurons, the resulting condition can be immovable, rigid musculature or immovable, flaccid musculature.

A pitta spike at majjā indicates demyelination of the nerve sheath, leading to multiple sclerosis. Pitta creates inflammation, neuritis or inflammatory conditions and eventually manifests as meningitis or encephalitis. These are serious conditions, but less serious are neuralgia and sciatica. Pitta in majjā dhātu can also create herpes zoster, which is an acute inflammation along the track of the nerve, or optic neuritis which precedes multiple sclerosis. If a person has pitta in majjā, it should be quickly treated, because it can lead to serious problems. On the level of the mind, pitta in majjā dhātu may create personality problems, such as schizophrenia. Take this condition seriously and cool down the pitta.

A kapha spike at the majjā dhātu position indicates hydrocephalus in children, which is increased intracranial pressure, and tumors in either the gray or white matter of the brain. A tumor in the white matter involves tarpaka kapha. Another condition is neurofibromatosis, a disease called elephant man syndrome because of the appearance created on the body. Excess kapha in majjā can also create hypersomnia, lethargy, depression and melancholia.

Shukra and Ārtava

When vāta is in shukra or ārtava, those dhātus become dry and debilitated. Men as well as women have menopause. Shukra dhātu is active in a man from age 16 to 70 and ārtava is active in a woman from age 12 until about age 50. Men after age 70 and women after 50 can commonly experience loss of energy in shukra and ārtava, leading to low libido. Vāta in shukra dhātu can lead to premature ejaculation in a man. In the same way, vāta in the ārtava manifests as menopause. If a woman has had a hysterectomy, the pulse will show vāta in the ārtava because of the creation of empty space.

A pitta spike at the shukra dhātu site may indicate a previous history of orchitis, epididymitis or prostatitis, or a family history of some prostate problem. Pitta in ārtava dhātu shows endometritis, fibroid tumor or multiple miscarriages. When there is excess pitta in ārtava, a woman may have sensitive nipples and tender breasts, and the high pitta can affect stanya (lactation). There is a functional relationship between ārtava and stanya. Other pitta-in-ārtava conditions include Bartholin's gland inflammation, cervicitis and cervical dysplasia, which is considered a pre-cancerous symptom. Pitta in ārtava dhātu can create oophoritis, leading to painful ovaries. In some individuals it may lead to vaginitis—which may be one of several types of infection in the vagina, including fungal infections and chlamydia.

A kapha spike at the site of shukra may indicate prostatic calculi, a testicular tumor, testicular swelling or hydrocele, which is an accumulation of water within the scrotal skin. This condition may also be due to pitta, if inflammation is present. Kapha in ārtava dhātu may manifest as an ovarian cyst or cystic ovary and pseudo-pregnancy. In that condition, the woman has a strong desire to become a mother but endometriosis blocks the tube and the woman develops a false pregnancy. The cells of the uterus lose their intelligence, thinking that the uterus has conceived, and continue to grow. This type of condition is known as gulma in Sanskrit. Sometimes vāta in ārtava can create an ectopic gestation or tubular pregnancy; however, this condition may also be due to a blockage by kapha. When kapha partially obstructs the tube, tubular pregnancy can occur.

EXAMPLES OF SPECIFIC DISEASES FOUND IN THE FIFTH LEVEL PULSE

Granthi Rūpa Nādi (Syphilitic Arteriosclerosis).

The pulse in this condition feels knotted, thickened and jerky, and recedes completely between beats. This is due to syphilitic arteriosclerosis, which is pitta in rakta dhātu.

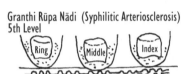

Granthi Rūpa Nādi (Syphilitic Arteriosclerosis)
5th Level

Upa Damsha (Syphilis).
If the pulse under the middle finger at the shukra or ārtava site on the fifth level has high tension and it curves and then slips off the finger, that denotes syphilis.

Upa Damsha (Syphilis)
5th Level

Granthi Roga (Lymphadenitis).
A pitta spike at the rasa dhātu site under the ring finger indicates lymphadenitis, which is inflammation of the lymph nodes. The pulse is full, slippery and stout.

Granthi Roga (Lymphadenitis)
5th Level

Pitta spike at Rasa Dhātu

Shlīpada (Elephantiasis of the Leg).
In *shlīpada*, elephantiasis of the leg, the pulse under the ring finger on both sides of the client at the fifth level rasa dhātu site shows a kapha spike. The pulse is slow, dull, full and depressed and is curved. There is solid, thick edema in both legs and they look like the legs of an elephant, as shown in the diagram.

Shlīpada
(Elephantiasis of the Leg)
5th Level

Visphota (Herpes Zoster or Shingles).
Herpes zoster is indicated by a strong pitta spike at the rakta dhātu site under the ring finger on the fifth level. Excess pitta in the blood can create hemorrhagic spots at the site of the breakout of shingles on the skin.

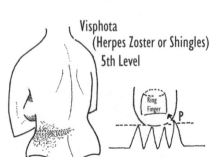

Visphota
(Herpes Zoster or Shingles)
5th Level

Visarpa (Erysipelas). Erysipelas is a contagious disease of the skin and subcutaneous tissues due to infection with Streptococcus pyogenes, with redness and swelling of affected areas and sometimes with vesicular lesions. The pulse under the ring finger at the rakta dhātu site of the fifth level is distressed, weak and slender with frequent jerks and moves slowly like a snake chasing a frog, i.e., vāta pushing pitta.

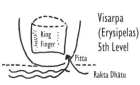

Visarpa

Visarpa
(Erysipelas)
5th Level

Ring Finger

Pitta

Rakta Dhātu

Ūrdhva Jatru Granthi (Hyperthyroidism). Hyperthyroidism manifests in the pulse as a strong pitta spike at the distal curvature of the ring finger of the rakta dhātu pulse. The pulse has an abrupt strong spike and is quite fast. There are tremors of the hands and tongue, the eyes are protruded and the thyroid gland is enlarged.

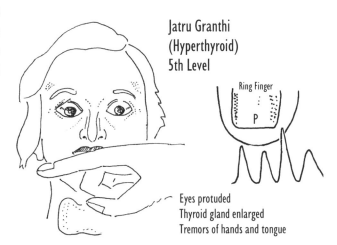

Jatru Granthi
(Hyperthyroid)
5th Level

Ring Finger

P

Eyes protuded
Thyroid gland enlarged
Tremors of hands and tongue

Asthi Saushiryam (Osteoporosis). A fast, thin, feeble pulse with an abrupt spike that moves like a cobra under the index finger at the asthi dhātu site is a sign of thin bones or osteoporosis. This condition manifests most frequently in old age and in post-menopausal women. A similar condition with a similar pulse is sometimes found in children at about the age of seven. This condition is called osteogenesis imperfecta. It is caused by congenital vāta in asthi dhātu manifesting as multiple fractures. As noted in the diagram, it creates a blue color to the sclera of the eye.

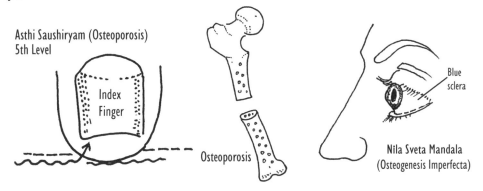

Asthi Saushiryam (Osteoporosis)
5th Level

Index
Finger

Osteoporosis

Blue
sclera

Nīla Sveta Mandala
(Osteogenesis Imperfecta)

Avabāhuka (Arthritis of the Shoulder Joint). In cases of acute arthritis of the shoulder joint, the pulse under the index finger at the asthi site becomes full and bounding. This pulse can be felt on the same side of the body as the arthritic lesion.

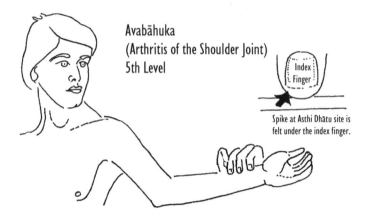

Avabāhuka
(Arthritis of the Shoulder Joint)
5th Level

Index Finger

Spike at Asthi Dhātu site is felt under the index finger.

Āma Vāta (Rheumatoid Arthritis). Rheumatoid arthritis creates muscle wasting, nodules and flexion deformities with joint swelling. A slender, heavy, abrupt cobra pulse is felt at the asthi and majjā sites under the index finger. Note the diagram of the eye showing recurrent scleritis with thinning of the sclera and glaucoma. A person with *āma vāta* usually has a history of rheumatic fever. This condition is caused by an autoimmune problem leading to āma in majjā dhātu. If the same pulse is felt only under the asthi dhātu site, that condition is called osteoarthritis (*sandhi vāta*) and is due to an autoimmune dysfunction of asthi dhātu.

Āma Vāta (Rheumatoid Arthritis)
5th Level

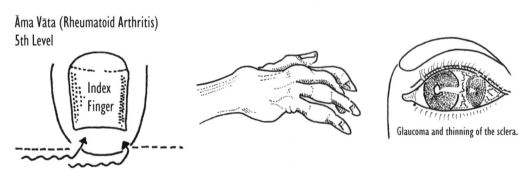

Index Finger

Glaucoma and thinning of the sclera.

Asthi Bhagna (Bone Fracture). The dhātu pulse under all three fingers is quick, feeble and cold to the touch. The asthi pulse has a strong vāta spike, which shows fracture of the shaft of a bone.

Urustambha (Paraplegia). In cases of paraplegia, the pulse under the index finger on both sides of the body is fast and feeble at the majjā dhātu site.

Urustambha (Paraplegia)
5th Level

Index Finger

Dhanustambha or Hanustambha (Tetanus or Lockjaw). In *dhanustambha* (tetanus), the fifth level pulse forcibly goes up and down and the spike is felt at the majjā dhātu site. In this illness, the body is rigidly fixed like a bow, as shown in the diagram. The retracted head is buried in the pillow, showing signs of meningeal irritation. In the case of *hanustambha* (lockjaw), the fifth level pulse becomes forceful at one moment and imperceptible at the next. The spike is felt at the site of majjā dhātu under the index finger.

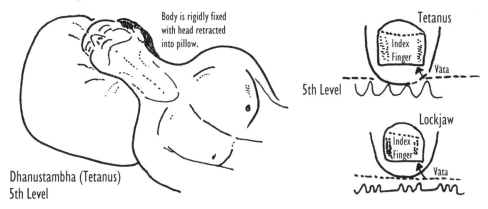

Body is rigidly fixed with head retracted into pillow.

Dhanustambha (Tetanus) 5th Level

Tetanus — Index Finger — Vāta — 5th Level

Lockjaw — Index Finger — Vāta

Vepathu (Parkinson's Disease). In cases of Parkinson's disease, the majjā dhātu pulse is hard, sclerosed and elongated, with a slow and low rise and fall. This pulse is slender and shows vāta characteristics. It is best felt under the index finger. This condition is called *vepathu* or *kampa vāta*. The patient has a typical masked-face appearance as shown in the diagram. Note the fixed stare, dribbling saliva and angular stomatitis. The body becomes stiff and the fingers make pill rolling movements.

Vepathu (Parkinson's Disease) 5th Level, Majja Dhātu Pulse

Index Finger — V

Parkinsonial face. Note the fixed stare, dribbling saliva and angular stomatitis.

Sūryāvarta (Migraine). The majjā dhātu site shows a strong jumping pitta spike, due to the heat created by high pitta, which causes the blood vessels to expand and press the nerves, causing pain.

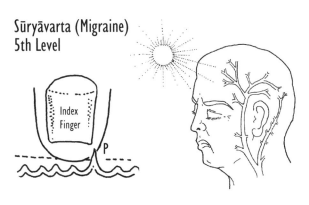

Sūryāvarta (Migraine) 5th Level

Index Finger — P

Garbhā Sravanam (Miscarriage or Abortion). In cases of miscarriage or abortion, the pulse under the middle finger shows a high pitta spike at the ārtava dhātu site, as shown in the diagram.

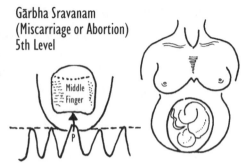

Gārbha Sravanam
(Miscarriage or Abortion)
5th Level

Pradara (Leukorrhea). The pradara pulse is slow and wavy and is best felt under the ring finger at the ārtava site, as shown in the diagram. This pulse has the deep and slow characteristics of kapha.

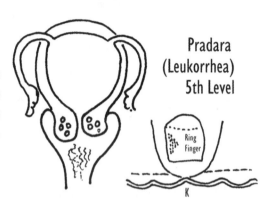

Pradara
(Leukorrhea)
5th Level

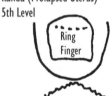

Kanda (Prolapsed Uterus)
5th Level

Kanda (Prolapsed Uterus). If the pulse under the ring finger at the ārtava site on both sides of the body is delicate, feeble and slow, it indicates a prolapsed uterus.

Soma Roga (Endometriosis). The ārtava dhātu pulse shows a deep, slow, wavy kapha pulse under the ring finger. This denotes a kapha disorder of ārtava vaha srotas. Due to excess kapha, the endometrial tissue grows outside the uterus into the abdominal and pelvic cavities.

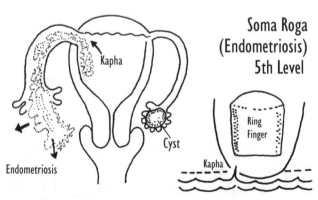

Soma Roga
(Endometriosis)
5th Level

OTHER ASPECTS OF THE FIFTH LEVEL PULSE

Samprāpti—The Process of Disease

An important and interesting aspect of the Āyurvedic pulse system relates to its ability to explain the pathogenesis of a disease. We have seen how vāta, pitta and kapha go out of balance and express this imbalance in a tissue, organ or system. According to this paradigm, each healthy, balanced dosha is at home in a particular area—vāta in the colon, pitta in the small intestine and kapha in the stomach. These are the primary sites of functioning from which the dosha can spread its influence.

How this happens is explained in a six stage model of pathogenesis called samprāpti. Accumulation (quantitatively) of the dosha marks the first stage of imbalance. In this stage, called *sañchaya*, vāta, pitta or kapha accumulates in its own site. Symptoms are usually mild, but the condition can be detected through the pulse even in this early stage. Using vāta for an example, high vāta in the colon would be experienced as gas and bloating. Aggravating influences might cause a further increase of vāta and qualitatively degrade its functioning, creating constipation and moving vāta to the second stage of aggravation or *prakopa*. In this stage, the doshic level rises in its own "container" in the body.

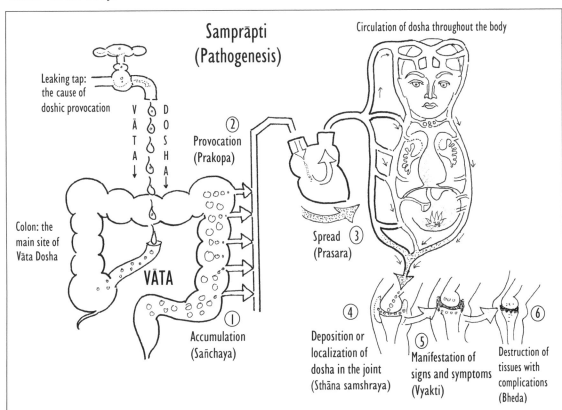

Samprāpti (Pathogenesis)

Circulation of dosha throughout the body

Leaking tap: the cause of doshic provocation

VĀTA ↓ DOSHA ↓

② Provocation (Prakopa)

Colon: the main site of Vāta Dosha

VĀTA

① Accumulation (Sañchaya)

③ Spread (Prasara)

④ Deposition or localization of dosha in the joint (Sthāna samshraya)

⑤ Manifestation of signs and symptoms (Vyakti)

⑥ Destruction of tissues with complications (Bheda)

Further aggravation escalates the situation to the third stage of spreading, called prasara. A dosha in this stage will leave the GI tract and enter the general circulation, "looking" for a place to enter. It will tend to move into a spot that has a weakness or defect, perhaps by virtue of a genetic flaw or some previous disease. Any aggravated dosha has an affinity for moving into these weak spots, called khavaigunya or defective space, which can be compared to potholes on a road.

On entering a tissue, the dosha influences the tissue by its aggravated qualities. Later, the dosha further invades the tissue and affects its functions. This amalgamation of dosha and dhātu is the stage of *sthāna samshraya*, stage four.

In the next stage, qualitative changes become apparent. The aggressive quality of dosha suppresses the natural quality of the dhātu, resulting in pathological conditions. For example, because of its cold quality, vāta can create stiffness in the joints. Due to its dry and rough qualities, vāta creates cracking and deformity of the articular surface. Because of the rough quality, vāta will create pain. This occurs in the fifth stage of manifestation, called *vyakti*. The subtle attributes of the dosha have by now totally manifested according to the etiological factors. One can not only label the illness but also point out the particular quality of the dosha that is playing the most important role in the disease process. In the vyakti stage, all functional changes become evident.

In stage six, called *bheda*, structural changes manifest. Complications involving other organs, tissues or systems also become evident. Vāta will not only affect the joint space but also the surrounding soft tissue, leading to muscle wasting, frozen joints and deformity. This stage is the final expression of the disease process. The disease has completely manifested with its complications and must be dealt with by effective means.

We have used vāta as an example for showing the disease process but the same progression is true for pitta and kapha. The pulse, by disclosing which doshas are involved and if any tissues and organs are affected, can reveal which stage of pathogenesis has been reached. The details of the dosha involved suggest the nature of a disorder in a particular tissue or organ. The fifth level dhātu pulses and deep and superficial level organ pulses divulge the specific sites where an imbalance is occurring and which doshas are affecting these tissues and organs. The pulses of the subtypes of the doshas give information about what is happening functionally in the areas of the body related to each subdosha.

संचयं च प्रकोपं च प्रसरं स्थानसंश्रयम् ।
व्यक्तिं भेदं च यो वेत्ति दोषाणां स भवेद्भिषक् ॥ ३६ ॥
सु. सू. २१

One who knows the various stages of pathogenesis—accumulation (sañchaya), provocation (prakopa), spread or diffusion (prasara), deposition or localization (sthāna samshraya), manifestation (vyakti) and the differentiation or termination (bheda)—is entitled to be a physician.

Su. Sū. 21:36

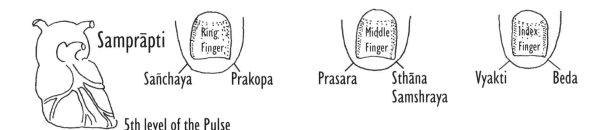

Samprāpti

Sañchaya   Prakopa   Prasara   Sthāna   Vyakti   Beda
                                   Samshraya

Ring Finger   Middle Finger   Index Finger

5th level of the Pulse

How to Feel Samprāpti in the Fifth Level Pulse. At the fifth level of the pulse, we can also precisely detect the stage of samprāpti. By bringing one's attention to this level, we can find out where there is a doshic spike. Each stage of samprāpti is reflected in its own site, on either the distal or proximal side of the central curvature of each finger, as shown in the diagram. These are the same positions as those used to assess the dhātus.

When *dosha sañchaya* happens, the qualities of any dosha currently in that stage are felt on the proximal side of the central curvature of the ring finger. This is the same site as that used to feel rasa dhātu. For instance, a spike with pitta qualities on the distal side of the ring finger indicates that pitta dosha is in the first stage of samprāpti, sañchaya. Prakopa is assessed on the distal side of the ring finger, the same position as the rakta spike. Prasara is felt by a spike at the site of māmsa dhātu, which is the proximal side of the curvature on the middle finger. Sthāna samshraya is ascertained at the distal position on the middle finger, which is also used for meda dhātu. Vyakti is read at the proximal curvature of the index finger, the asthi site, and finally bheda can be felt on the distal side of the index finger, in the majjā dhātu position.

As an example, if there is a vāta spike on the distal side of the middle finger, it shows that vāta is in the fourth stage of sthāna samshraya. Likewise, if a kapha spike is felt on the proximal side of the index finger, that means kapha is in the fifth stage—vyakti. To sense these qualities, one needs a great deal of sensitive awareness. Such sensitivity gives us a great deal of useful information about the state of samprāpti. Hence we can use the fifth level pulse not only to find out the state of each dhātu, but to ascertain the current stage of samprāpti for each of the three doshas.

Pregnancy

Pregnancy can be detected in the fifth level of a woman's pulse, at the site of ārtava dhātu. If the nādi shifts toward either the lateral side (the thumb side or radial border) or medial side (the little finger side or ulnar border), it indicates the woman is pregnant. This pulse can be felt on both the right and left arms. A spike is different from a shift, because a spike goes up and down, whereas a shift moves horizontally. The feel of the

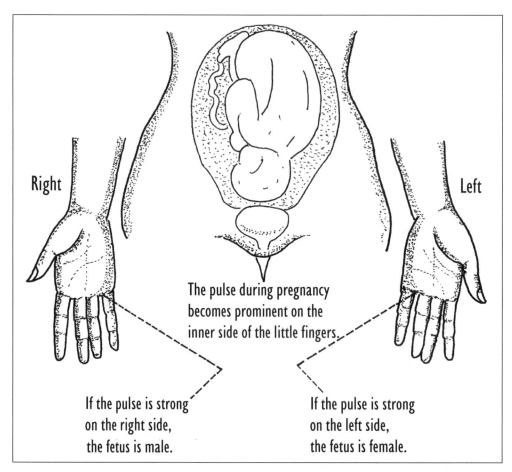

Right

Left

The pulse during pregnancy
becomes prominent on the
inner side of the little fingers.

If the pulse is strong
on the right side,
the fetus is male.

If the pulse is strong
on the left side,
the fetus is female.

ārtava pulse is different in case of pregnancy. For instance, if there is a disorder of vāta and there is no pregnancy, there will be a spike under the index finger, but there will be no shift. If the nāḍi shifts laterally, it indicates a male fetus, while a medial shift indicates a female fetus. This pulse can be felt within 15 to 30 days after conception, so the ārtava pulse is important for early detection of pregnancy.

While taking the pulse of a pregnant woman, pay complete attention and count to twelve vegas or beats. Within twelve vegas, the number of times the pulse shifts to a different direction will help to detect the time of conception. Within twelve beats the pulse will shift either to the outer or inner border. If it shifts once, it is the first month of pregnancy. If it shifts twice, it is the second month of pregnancy; if three times, it is the third month; and so on. If it is twins, the pulse will shift to both sides—outside and inside. The number of beats between shifts represents the number of days since ovulation. Being able to perceive these shifts depends upon clear perception and sensitive awareness.

During a shift, if there is an interruption of the pitta or vāta spikes, it signifies miscarriage, obstructed labor or placenta previa. If the gati under the kapha and pitta fingers is regular without the interruption of the pitta or vāta spikes, it denotes a smooth, normal delivery. A shift under the vāta finger shows the woman has been pregnant for a short period of time and there is a *gandakāla* (indication of critical illness) to the fetus. A vāta spike under the kapha finger denotes ovulation.

To detect the unborn child's prakruti, go to the fifth level and focus one's attention at the central part of the fingers. If the shift occurs under the index finger, the child's prakruti is vāta. A shift under the middle finger indicates pitta prakruti. If the shifting is under the ring finger, the child's constitution is predominantly kapha. If shifting is felt under two fingers, the child's constitution is dual doshic, such as vāta-pitta or pitta-kapha equally predominant.

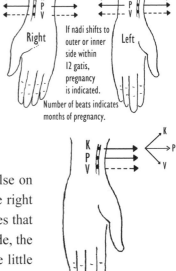

There is also another way to confirm pregnancy. Feel the pulse on the lateral or inner side at the base of the little finger, on both the right and left hands. If the pulse at this location is prominent, it indicates that conception has taken place. If it is more prominent on the right side, the fetus is male. If it is more prominent on the left side, female. The little finger pulse is a confirmative test. This pulse also indicates ovulation. If the spike is strong and the woman is not pregnant, the indication is ovulation.

Remember that we are feeling the pulse at the fifth level at the ārtava dhātu location for a minimum of twelve beats. Within those twelve beats, if there is a horizontal shift, a pregnancy is indicated. If the shift is to the outside, toward the radial bone of the client, the conceived fetus is male. If the shift is to the inside, toward the ulnar bone, the conceived fetus is female. How can we distinguish this pulse from ārtava vikruti? Vikruti doesn't shift; it will give only an upward spike with the characteristics of vāta, pitta or kapha.

Gandakāla in the Fifth Level Pulse

In between the astral body and physical body there is a subtle channel called chitrā nādi, which is expressed in the fifth level of the pulse. The events of gandakāla come to the physical level through *chitrā nādi*. Gandakāla means an indication or warning of a future critical illness or accident. It may not be a pathological condition that will manifest; it may not even be a psychological condition. It may be a spiritual event or an astral occurrence that will happen to the person. This indication or warning of the future is felt only in the fifth level pulse. This pulse shows how we bridge intelligence and intuition, as the knowledge gained from this pulse comes from intuition. I am talking about something beyond logic and that which is beyond logic is difficult to put into words.

Irregular gati within 12 beats indicates gandakāla.

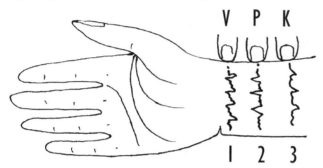

To find the gandakāla pulse, once again go to the fifth level at the shukra/ārtava location. This pulse is entirely different from the other pulses we have discussed at the fifth level. The gandakāla pulse indicates a vulnerable time during which some sickness or serious event may happen. It indicates a need to change the diet and lifestyle, and to rest, read and relax. It is important to know this pulse. It gives expression of movement in the nādi, revealing that there is order in chaos. We can tune into these deep and pervading cycles of influence and give a warning bell to the person. There may not actually be any current pathology. The gandakāla may be connected karmically to the astral body and may manifest later as illness or accident, but something is going to occur.

An irregular rhythm under the vāta finger (index finger) within 12 beats denotes gandakāla within approximately six months. An irregular rhythm under the pitta finger (middle finger) within 12 beats indicates gandakāla within three months. Irregular gati under the kapha finger (ring finger) means that within one month there will be a gandakāla. Remember that this pulse is felt at the ārtava / shukra location, but it has nothing to do with the dhātu.

The critical time for gandakāla at each pulse location is:

✧ within six months if detected under the vāta finger
✧ within three months if found under the pitta finger
✧ within one month if discovered under the kapha finger

There is another method of taking this pulse. Suppose you are sitting facing the person. "Look" directly into the third eye of that person and then feel your own pulse. As you tune in with that person, you start feeling that person's pulse in your own. That is called tele-pulse and it can also be done at a distance.

Summary

I have shared with you what to see, when to see it and how to feel it. You have to practice on your own pulse, reading all seven levels. You will learn by self-observation. Then also read the pulses of family members to gain more experience. After reading hundreds of pulses, new centers are sensitized at the tips of the fingers and through those centers you will develop different doors of perception. It takes the examination of a minimum of one thousand pulses in order to develop these skills of tactile perception.

Āyurveda, to a certain extent, is a science. It is logic, it has philosophy, anatomy and physiology, pharmacology, and so forth as well as diagnostic techniques such as pulse reading, inspection, palpation and percussion. In this chapter, we have gone into other realms, which show that Āyurveda also has great spirituality and a profound mystic quality that can lead to highly developed intuition. When one learns Āyurveda, one's life will be changed. One will start thinking in terms of the beyond, in terms of the immeasurable and the unknown. The unknown is not unknowable. It is in the subconscious, while the known is conscious. The meeting point of the unknown and the known is the meeting of the conscious and subconscious, where there is a door to the superconscious. In the superconscious state, the unknown becomes knowable.

PRĀNA, TEJAS, OJAS
The Subtle, Refined Essences of the Tissues
Level Four

सत्त्वमात्मा शरीरं च त्रयमेतत्त्रिदण्डवत् ।
लोकस्तिष्ठति संयोगत्तत्र सर्वं प्रतिष्ठितम् ॥ ४६ ॥
च. सू. १

*The body, mind and soul exist together as one
unit (the tripod of life), as all things in the
universe exist together in harmony.*

Ca. Sū. 1:46

Inside the white matter of the brain there is space. There are small spaces between neurons called synaptic spaces. This synaptic space is functionally connected to the space within the brain called chidākāsha. Within that space is a pulsation of prāna and a flow of ojas and tejas.

Prāna carries sensation through the vagus and phrenic nerves into the cardiac plexus. In Sanskrit, pulsation is called prāna spanda. Spanda, which is the pranic current from the hypothalamus to the heart, moves at intervals of .08 seconds and stimulates the pacemaker sinoatrial node, the SA node, which is present in the right atrium. From there, the pranic stimulation is carried down to the AV (atrioventricular) node. Thus prāna regulates the movements of the heart.

The heart is a type of battery. In its rhythmic movement, the heart generates electricity that is carried through the blood vessels and even to the skin. This movement of cardiac activity can be traced with a sensitive galvanometer. So pulse not only represents the heart pumping, it also represents the flow of prāna and vyāna vāyu.

In this chapter we will switch our attention to the fourth level of the pulse, which is the level of prāna, tejas and ojas. Ojas is the pure essence of all dhātus (tissues) and is produced during the process of nutrition. It can be compared to the modern concept of

हृदि तिष्ठति यच्छुद्धं रक्तमीषत्सपीतकम् ।
ओजः शरीरे संख्यातं तन्नाशान्ना विनश्यति ॥ ७४ ॥

The white, yellowish-red fluid that lodges in
the heart is called ojas (the refined essence
of all tissues of the body). If it is lost, the
person dies.

प्रथमं जायते ह्योजः शरीरेऽस्मिञ्छरीरिणाम् ।
सर्पिर्वर्णं मधुरसं लाजगन्धि प्रजायते ॥ ७५ ॥
च. सू. १७

Ojas (vital essence) is the first thing created
in the body of all living beings. Its color is like
ghee, it tastes like honey and smells like
roasted puffed rice.

Ca. Sū. 17:74-75

albumin. Ojas includes albumin but albumin alone is not ojas. Ojas also includes protein and globulin, which are necessary to maintain immunity. But to say that these three are ojas also doesn't convey the entire meaning. Ojas is not an abstract concept but is an actual substance.

Āyurveda has described two types of ojas. Inferior ojas is half an *añjali* in quantity (see Glossary). It moves throughout the body. Superior ojas is eight drops in quantity, and it stays in the heart. This ojas has the smell of *ghee* and rice. It is yellowish-white in color, cool in attribute and tastes like honey. Ojas moves through the plasma and is represented at the fourth level by the pulsation under the ring finger, the kapha finger.

Tejas can be compared to hormones and amino acids. There are 21 or more important amino acids that regulate cellular metabolism. Tejas is necessary for *pīlu pāka* and *pithara pāka*, the agnis of cellular and nuclear metabolism. Tejas is also responsible for intelligence, understanding and comprehension at the cellular level. It is felt under the middle finger at the fourth level.

Every cell is a center of awareness and consciousness and every cell is a unit of life. At one time, each of us was an atomic cell. From that one cell, the sperm and ovum develop into a complex multi-cellular mammal. There is a continuous flow of intelligence and communication between the cells of the body, called prāna. The prāna spike is found under the index finger at the fourth level. Prāna is the essence of vāta; tejas is the essence of pitta; and ojas is the pure essence of kapha.

If the fourth level pulse is slow, cold and deep, it indicates feeble prāna, tejas or ojas, depending on which finger is affected. In a normal and healthy condition, the seventh level of prakruti and the fourth level of prāna-tejas-ojas should show the same

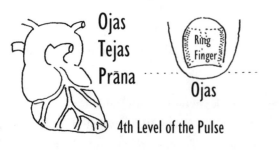

Ojas
Tejas
Prāna

Ojas

4th Level of the Pulse

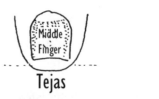

Tejas

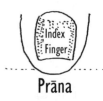

Prāna

reading, with the same number of spikes in the same respective positions. For instance, a person with a prakruti pulse of $V_1 P_2 K_3$ should have a fourth level pulse of Prāna$_1$ Tejas$_2$ Ojas$_3$ ($P_1 T_2 O_3$). In other words, the prāna reading at the fourth level should match the vāta reading in the prakruti pulse, the tejas should be the same as pitta in the prakruti, and ojas the same as for kapha in the deep level pulse. If the prakruti pulse and the fourth level pulse differ, this indicates a disorder of prāna, tejas or ojas. It may be increased raw prāna, tejas or ojas, or it could be low prāna, tejas or ojas.

When feeling the pulse, use the right arm for a male and the left for a female, and gently touch the superficial skin and feel the throbbing at the first level. Go down slightly and feel the spike change at the second level. Then at the third level the spike changes again. With delicate pressure go to the fourth level, where the spike once again changes. At that level, feel the strength and quality of the spike. A spike under the kapha finger denotes the strength of ojas. The middle finger shows the power of tejas and the index finger indicates the strength of prāna. When the spike is weak, prāna is weak; when the spike is strong, prāna is strong. In the same way, if the spike under the middle finger is feeble, tejas is low; if the spike is strong, tejas is strong.

To detect these differences is subjective. Three plus (+++) is good ojas. Two plus (++) is moderate ojas. One plus (+) is low ojas. One plus is 25 percent, two plus 50 percent, three plus 100 percent. One hundred percent superfine quality of ojas is present in a perfectly healthy individual. However, we work hard, we have troubling emotions and we have responsibilities, and all these stresses deplete ojas.

In certain AIDS patients, a very feeble ojas pulse is present, because their ojas is depleted. If tejas is four plus, that indicates high (raw) tejas, which burns ojas. For example, in multiple sclerosis, the myelin sheath, which is composed of ojas, is being burned by high tejas. Therefore, there is demyelination occurring, which leads to multiple sclerosis. That is why patients of multiple sclerosis are exhausted when exposed to too much cold or hot weather. Both heat and cold bother them because four plus tejas is abnormal. Four plus ojas is high (raw) ojas, which creates diabetes and may lead to high cholesterol and high triglycerides. High (raw) prāna makes a person hyperactive and anxious.

TREATMENT OF DEPLETED PRĀNA

In order to improve prāna, do prānāyāma. *Nādi shodana,* alternate nostril breathing, is a good form of beginning prānāyāma. Sit comfortably on the floor in a cross-legged posture. If you are not comfortable in this position, then sit upright on the front edge of a chair with your feet flat on the floor. Close the right nostril with the right thumb and inhale gradually through the left nostril into the belly, not into the chest. On inhalation, count 1-2-3-4. After a full inhalation, close both the nostrils and do a gentle chin lock as you hold the breath in the belly and count 1-2-3-4, up to 16. Use a count of 4 to inhale and 16 to retain. Then open the right nostril while holding the left nostril closed with the ring and little fingers and exhale through the right nostril while counting to 8. The exhalation should be slow and steady as you count 1-2-3-4-5-6-7-8. The speed of the counting should be equal, with a count of 4 for inhalation, 16 for retention, and 8 for exhalation. If this approach is too complicated or difficult at first, then inhale only for 2, retain up to 8, and exhale for 4 counts. After exhalation from the right nostril, hold the breath outside for awhile, then inhale through the right nostril, hold the breath into the belly by closing both nostrils, and then exhale through the left nostril. Repeat, alternating the nostrils through which you inhale.

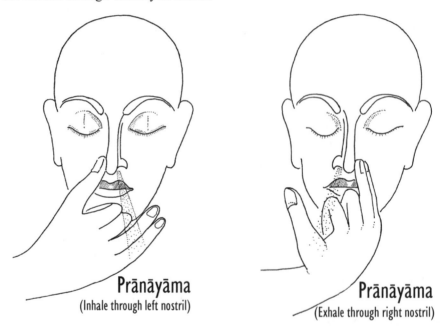

Prāṇāyāma
(Inhale through left nostril)

Prāṇāyāma
(Exhale through right nostril)

If the mind is too busy with the counting, just inhale slowly into the belly through the left nostril by closing the right nostril. After a full inhalation, close both nostrils and do a chin lock. Place your total attention behind the belly button. When oxygen is depleted in the lungs, one gets a swallowing reflex, which is the sign to exhale. Then slowly exhale through the opposite nostril. During exhalation, there should be a continuous slow flow, as you let the air dissolve into the outer space. Stay outside for a moment, then inhale through the right nostril, retain, and exhale through the left. Then inhale through the left, retain, and exhale through the right; and so forth. During breath retention, do a chin lock, and during exhalation release that lock. Use the chin lock to avoid direct pressure in the brain through the carotid artery. Do five rounds of this prāṇāyāma, rest for one minute, then again do five more rounds. In this way, the vital capacity of the lungs can be increased. This prāṇāyāma, as well as the others in this book, are best learned from an accomplished teacher.

Another prāṇāyāma is *bhastrikā,* the breath of fire. In this prāṇāyāma, inhalation is passive, but exhalation is active, with a little force. Start slowly, then increase the speed. Imagine a steam engine moving slowly and then gradually increasing the train speed. This action is a form of thoraco-abdominal hyperventilation. Do one round of 30 strokes or exhalations, then rest for one minute. This prāṇāyāma also increases the vital capacity of the lungs. Practice five rounds of bhastrikā in the morning and five rounds in the evening. It will help to relieve allergy and asthma, making the lungs strong and healthy. Don't do bhastrikā during menstruation or pregnancy and if your pitta is high, substitute *shītali,* a cooling prāṇāyāma that involves breathing through a curled tongue.

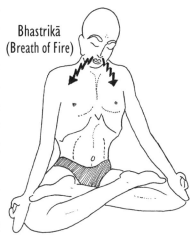

Bhastrikā
(Breath of Fire)

Another good prāṇāyāma is called *bhrāmarī* (humming). On inhalation, constrict the epiglottis and create a humming sound. On exhalation, the sound becomes long and low. The inhalation is like the sound of a female bee and the exhalation is like the sound of a male bee. If it is difficult to create a humming noise during inhalation, just inhale naturally, take a breath deep into the belly, do a chin lock and then do bhrāmarī on the exhale. Bhrāmarī improves the melody of the voice. In addition, the humming vibrates the nervous system and is a form of sound therapy for the brain. Bhrāmarī is also good for the thyroid, thymus and parathyroid glands. When doing bhrāmarī, touch the tip of the tongue to the edge of the soft palate, near the back of the roof of the mouth, and be sure the teeth are not clenched. The pineal gland is stimulated by touching the tip of the tongue to the soft palate near the uvula. Chemoreceptors are present on the mucous membrane of the palate that stimulate the secretion of serotonin and melatonin. In addition, placing the tongue in this position also helps to secrete soma. Soma, a mystical substance that is sometimes called the divine nectar, brings tranquility and nourishes ojas, tejas and prāna, because soma is the mother of these three.

Hummmmm
Hummmm

Bhrāmarī Prāṇāyāma
(with chin lock and
humming breathing)

Sit in the lotus pose for meditation. Each knee represents a petal of the lotus. Pressure comes directly to the tip of the spine and the whole vertebral column remains straight. With persistent practice, one can easily sit in a lotus pose for one, two or even three hours and, if one sits properly in a lotus pose for three hours each day, enlightenment will soon come. Sitting in the lotus pose helps to open the heart chakra, breathing becomes quiet, and ojas, tejas and prāna become balanced. Thinking stops automatically and thought cannot come, even if one decides to think. To go beyond thought is to go beyond suffering, because thought creates suffering.

Bhairavī mudrā, also called *shāmbhavī mudrā,* is very powerful. It expands the right and left ventricles of the brain and opens the chidākāsha, the space of awareness. Shāmbhavī refers to Shambu, another name of Lord Shiva. In this state, prāna is enhanced. One can strengthen prāna with prānāyāma through bhrāmarī and bhastrikā, whereas intense prāna unfolds in the lungs and body through bhairavī or shāmbhavī. One who fully practices shāmbhavī will be in a state of living samādhi. When practicing the bhairavī mudrā, one looks at any object, say a wall. When looking at the object, let the eyes look and do not blink the eyelids. The eyes are looking, yet the eyes are not looking, which means there is no judgment, no recognition, no identification. In Hindu art, philosophy and music, everything is a way to God-realization. Hindu philosophy includes the Vedas, Āyurveda, music, art and even dance. Everything is a movement of life. Therefore, the Hindu concept of God is *satyam shivam sundaram. Satyam* is the truth, shiva the holy and divine, and *sundaram* is beauty. Bhairavī manifests as satyam shivam sundaram.

As one looks outside, suddenly the attention goes inside. At that moment, an expansion of consciousness takes place. One is looking outside but the entire attention is inside, into the center of existence. In that state, one finds union with expansive consciousness. One looks around, but there is no choice in the looking, no judgment; just choiceless observation. In this sense, the choosers are the losers. The confused mind chooses. The mind that is insecure, agitated and unsatisfied chooses. Please don't misunderstand me; I am talking here about a different level of consciousness. In this art of meditation, choice has no place. Choice only has a place in the sense that one has chosen this way of meditation, that's all.

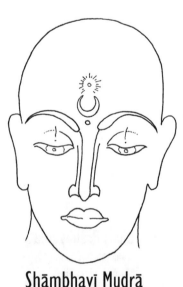

Shāmbhavī Mudrā

Look at anything, but in that looking there is emptiness. Thinking stops, breathing becomes quiet and one simply exists as pure awareness. In that state there is great joy, beauty and love. Sit absolutely relaxed, with no tension, and just look at the wall.

Slightly open the mouth with no expression on the face. The hands are like an empty bowl facing the sky. Simply look and allow the breathing to become quiet. Enlightenment can come in a fraction of a second. Samādhi means equilibrium. In that state, individual consciousness merges with cosmic consciousness and one goes beyond time and thought. In that state, whether the eyes are open or closed doesn't matter. It comes like a breeze, without invitation, because this state is your true nature—love, bliss, beauty and awareness. There is no fear, no depression, no anxiety, no worry, no stress. One becomes the witness of anxieties, worries and stress. In that state, healing occurs.

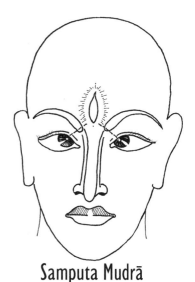

Samputa Mudrā

Gazing at the point between the eyebrows, the seat of the "third eye", strengthens insight and improves concentration on the inner flame of awareness.

There is another mudrā, called *samputa mudrā,* in which awareness becomes pinpointed and sharp. It opens the third eye and stills the mind. All of these mudrās indirectly help to balance ojas, tejas and prāna.

Practicing these prānāyāmas and mudrās every day will strengthen prāna and help one to move into an expansive state of consciousness. In that state, one loves everything—flowers, rocks, birds and trees. A stage will come in bhairavī where one feels "I am the sun; I am the star; I am the sky; I am the flower." This unity consciousness is bhakti, the love divine. Love and bhakti go together. To realize God is so simple, but man has tortured himself. It is good to have discipline, but one should do fasting, cleansing, *yoga* and prānāyāma without torture. In that way, these practices become spontaneous and natural and they will balance ojas, tejas and prāna.

TREATMENT OF DEPLETED TEJAS AND OJAS

Depleted ojas can be treated with almond milk. Soak 10 almonds in a cup of water overnight. In the morning, peel off the skins and put the almonds in a blender, adding one cup of hot milk. If the person is allergic to milk, use soy or rice milk. Add one teaspoon of date sugar, a pinch of cardamom, a pinch of ginger powder and one teaspoon of ghee and blend together. Regular brown sugar, sucanat or turbinado may be used instead of date sugar. Saffron may also be added, as well as a few drops of rose essence. This is a wonderful, rich drink to take in the morning to build ojas, and this drink is also good for building shukra after having sex. If cholesterol is a concern, use skim milk. Ghee increases the good cholesterol, called HDL, but if one's total cholesterol is high, don't take ghee.

For depleted tejas use one pinch of trikatu, which is a combination of ginger, black pepper, and long pepper (Piper longum or pippalī), and one teaspoon of honey. Take this combination about 15 minutes before lunch and dinner. These herbs taken before food kindle agni and act as an appetizer and digestive. Chewing a small piece of ginger with a pinch of salt and a few drops of fresh lime juice before eating will also kindle jāthara agni, thereby building tejas.

By using certain Ayurvedic herbal formulae, one can also improve prāna. Pippalī (long pepper) with honey and ghee is a specific *rasāyana* for prāna. Taking one-fourth teaspoon of triphala with one teaspoon each of honey and ghee in the early morning will help to create balance of prāna, tejas and ojas. There should be no fear of increasing cholesterol, because honey aids the regulation of cholesterol. In addition, shāmbhavī mudrā (*see* page 100) helps to balance ojas, tejas and prāna.

To build ojas one can take ghee, whereas castor oil is beneficial for vāta and, therefore, good for prāna. But to build up tejas, castor oil would not be a good idea. Bitter ghee (*tikta ghrita*) is good for tejas, because it enhances tejas but doesn't increase pitta. Take one teaspoon on an empty stomach twice a day, morning and evening, followed by half a cup of warm water.

BALANCING PRĀNA, TEJAS AND OJAS

Every thought is an electrical impulse. Every heart beat is an electrical impulse of prāna. The pericardium, along with the muscles of the heart, is a powerful electric generator and the electricity is maintained by ojas. During orgasm, one throws out energy from the body in the form of orgasmic fluid. So, for the sake of the heart and pericardium, reduce sexual activity or observe celibacy. Celibacy transforms that electricity into intelligence (tejas) and that intelligence becomes the aura. Kirlian photography reveals the auric picture and after sex, the aura is distorted and weakened. New life is created after intercourse and the purpose of sex is the creation of progeny. In the woman the orgasmic fluids contain ojas, so the woman also loses ojas (energy) due to excessive sexual activity. In tantra there is intercourse without ejaculation and, through yogic discipline, the sexual energy can be transformed into supreme intelligence. This sexual practice is not the suppression of the urge to have sex. However, there is danger in practicing tantra without proper guidance from a teacher.

We all need healing. We, as individuals, must bring awareness to our feelings and emotions. Otherwise, we never take responsibility for our healing. We always hold another person responsible for our suffering—mother, father or some planets in the sky. We need to accept the responsibility that "I am the pain and the pain is me. My pain is my creation; it is my reflection; it is me." We must understand our relationship with our suffering and, in that understanding, we maintain our ojas. In that ojas there is the beautiful light of tejas, which is the perception. And in the flame of attention, grief and sadness burn and we become totally free.

We have to protect our prāna, tejas and ojas through awareness, because awareness is the flame of attention, the luminosity of tejas. Prāna directs attention to something, creating perception. Attention plus prāna is perception. There are many things waiting for our perception, but we cannot perceive everything at one time. Perception is a product of time and our perception is a learned phenomenon, which is directed by knowledge and experience. In the perception of observer, object and observation, this trinity becomes one when prāna, tejas and ojas are balanced. This balanced state is perfect health.

When we are honest with our feelings and emotions, ojas is building, tejas is glowing, and prāna is flowing. That is a state of good health, existing at every moment, in every event of life. Āyurveda says every breath, every moment, every event should be lived with total awareness. When listening to someone, at the same time listen to the listener. When looking at an object, at the same moment look at the looker. When you look at me, my body is an object and you are the observer. When I am looking at you, your body is the object and I am the observer.

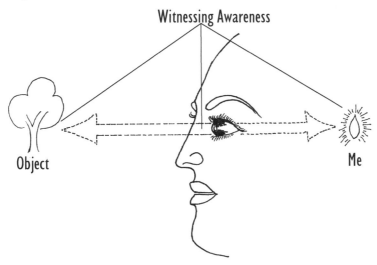

When you look outside, something like an arrow goes outwards. At the same time, a second arrow of attention goes into the heart, to look at the looker. This is called double-arrowed attention. In double-arrowed attention, a third phenomenon occurs, which is called witnessing. If you remain in witnessing, you will never get hurt. Forget about your past life. Forget about your future life. Your past life is recorded in your astral body. When practicing this awareness, that light, that flame, that fire of witnessing attention will burn. It will relieve the memory of parents' illnesses and past life hurt as well as suffering from this life. Just take responsibility, sit and meditate and do it. Unless you open your heart, unless you jump into the inner abyss, you are not going to become enlightened. Ultimately, you have to knock on your own door; you have to beg at your own door; you have to come back to yourself. Love is within you. God is within you.

Learning is sharing; it is a journey and an investigation together. Every morning upon waking, feel your own pulse. Now feel the pulse, bringing all tanmātrās to the tips of the fingers. Be your own healer, be your own doctor, be your own vaidya, and start reading your pulse. In that way, new centers will be created on the tips of the fingers, and those centers will become receptors through which information is received. As your finger receptors become more finely tuned and you continue to study your own pulse, your awareness will be raised and healing will come to you.

The relationship between teacher and taught is sacred and, once the student understands, it stays with him or her. Each student will learn Āyurveda from perception, experience and insight. When insight comes, the light within becomes visible. There is no light other than pure perception. That light, the guru within you, never dies. This guru is not a body; it is not a person; it is pure awareness, pure light, pure perception. Gu means darkness and ru means light, the light that dispels the darkness of ignorance. This knowledge comes from the pure consciousness of the master and the master is within you. That is the beauty of Āyurveda.

MANAS PRAKRUTI AND VIKRUTI
The Mental Constitution and
the Present Flow of Consciousness

Levels Six and Two

We have been learning the ancient art of feeling the pulse and have considered together the first (superficial) and seventh (deep) levels, as well as the third, fourth and fifth levels. Now we will shift our attention to *manas prakruti* and *manas vikruti*, which are found at the sixth and second levels.

Manas means mind. The mental and physical bodies are bridged together by prāna, the life force. Consciousness is the spirit or soul, about which modern medical science speaks very little. Because modern medical science places more emphasis on objective proof, it often overlooks subjectivity. The Sanskrit word *pratyaksham* means what one observes or perceives. Personal perception is limited and it is difficult to prove everything objectively. Subjectivity and objectivity must be bridged. Subjective experiences belong to the mind and objective barometers are connected to the body. Objectivity is limited, whereas subjective experiences are vast. For this reason, it is important to consider manas prakruti and vikruti, which form a bridge between objectivity and subjectivity.

Āyurveda is a science (objective truth), a philosophy (subjective truth) and an art of medicine. It assays the mental, physical, emotional and spiritual components of life—encompassing a complete definition of life. What emerges from this definition is the understanding that life expresses in these numerous modes and its influences upon us will affect all these aspects of life. Āyurveda holds that a mental trauma, for example, will have emotional, physical and spiritual implications. Each aspect of life both effects and reflects changes in the other modes of existence.

The sixth level of the pulse is related to the mental constitution. According to Charaka, mind is the faculty that directs the senses toward an object of perception, and then it carries the sensation to the intellect, to produce knowledge. Charaka also speaks about the pervasiveness of mind. Perception is a function of mind and all five tanmātrās are present both within and outside of the mind. The mind communicates with these subtle forces of the tanmātrās and, therefore, the mind also pervades everything.

Every object in this world is waiting for our perception, but unless we pay attention to these objects, they do not exist for us. Unless the mind directs the senses to a particular object, we cannot perceive it. Touch is a tanmātrā of the inner mind. The moment an outer object is touched, the mind carries that touch sensation to the inner faculty for interpretation. The same is true for the other four senses.

Perception is of three types—*sattvic, rajasic, tamasic*. Sattvic perception is pure, giving us knowledge that nourishes consciousness. The cell is a center of consciousness that is nourished by pure knowledge given by the mind. However, if the mind has more rajasic or tamasic qualities, perception is distorted, which builds up wrong conclusions, judgment, incorrect knowledge and false images. These distortions build āma and affect the individual psychosomatically.

We will now try to understand the flow of consciousness at the sixth level of the pulse. When checking the manas prakruti pulse, have the person sit facing the east. This position will help to clarify the reading. The lotus at the bottom of the illustration represents a finger resting on the radial artery. Under each finger that is checking the pulse, one can imagine that there is an eight-petaled lotus. When feeling someone's pulse, use the diagram of this lotus to find the locations of the spike under each finger. Each petal can be numbered for convenience

Manas Prakruti

Fire
Air
Water
Earth
Space

E
Vāta ♪
Pitta △
Kapha ☐
Indra
NE
Ishanya
Kubera
N
Vāyavya
Varuna
NW
W
SW
Agni
Yama
Nairutya
SE
S
8
1
2
7
3
6
5
4

1) Indra - Royal, religious
2) Agni - Knowledgeable, judgmental
3) Yama - Introspective, impartial, lonely, sad, grieving
4) Nairutya - Dull, sleepy, gloomy, sad, depressed
5) Varuna - Compassionate
6) Vāyavya - Emotional, with mood swings
7) Kubera - Wealthy, long-lived
8) Ishanya - Spiritual, fortunate

of understanding and the number of the petal where one feels a spike should be noted for each finger. One must use subtle awareness when feeling this sixth level pulse to perceive the location of each spike. For example, under the index (V) finger, one might note the direction as V_2. The middle (P) finger might indicate P_3. The ring (K) finger may reveal a reading of K_7.

The finger on which a spike is felt relates to the doshic influence on the deity characteristics. The qualities of these eight deities are expressed through the three doshas. For instance, Indra (petal number one) always indicates a royal and religious mind. However an Indra spike on the index finger (vāta) means the mind is religious but fear oriented, whereby the person is fearful of God and will follow a religion through fear. Whereas on the middle finger (pitta), an Indra spike indicates a religious nature with a desire for fame. Finally, an Indra spike on the ring finger (kapha) indicates that the person is religious, humble and generous. The various combinations of the three doshas and eight deities is shown in the table.

Table 7: Eight Deity Personalities and the Three Doshas

DEITY	ELEMENT	VĀTA INDEX FINGER	PITTA MIDDLE FINGER	KAPHA RING FINGER
INDRA	Water	Fear of God	Gives donations with name attached	Religious, gives anonymous donations
AGNI	Fire	Quick to know, but quick to forget	Competitive	Knowledge, forgiveness
YAMA	Earth	Fear of unknown	Frustration	Grief leads to surrender
NAIRUTYA	Fire and Air	Worthlessness, interrupted sleep	Gloomy, irritable during sleep	Deep dreamless sleep, depression
VARUNA	Water	Compassion of short duration	Compassion with desire for power	Compassion as a passion for all
VĀYAVYA	Air	Mood swings	Hate and jealousy	Prolonged, slow, sustained emotions
KUBERA	Water and Earth	Wealthy, with fear of thieves	Desires prestigious wealth	Wealth with humility and simplicity
ISHĀNYA	Space	Spiritually excited, exhibitionist	Righteous indignation, fanaticism	Authentically spiritual, keeping it unexposed

These are characteristics that can manifest in someone's personality if the spike of a particular petal is felt on each of the three fingers.

If the spike is felt in the position of petal number one (the east), that indicates an Indra personality, which is royal, religious and sattvic. If the spike is felt at the second petal (southeast), it shows an Agni personality, which relates to knowledge and rajas. That person is a worshipper of knowledge. The third petal (south) is a Yama personality, who is impartial and tamasic. Yama is the god of death, who takes away the soul and puts an end to the individual's life. He loves all equally. People with Yama personalities are quite impartial; they love no one, which means they love everyone, and they are also sad and introspective. A spike in the fourth petal position (southwest) indicates a Nairutya personality. These people love to sleep and are tamasic.

A spike in petal number five (west) shows Varuna, which is sattvic. People with a Varuna personality are loving and compassionate. Petal six (northwest) is Vāyavya, which is rajasic. The Vāyavya personality is emotional with mood swings. A spike at the seventh petal (north) indicates Kubera, which is sattvic. People with this pulse are rich in mind and blessed with long life. Petal eight (northeast) is Ishānya, which is also sattvic. These people are fortunate and spiritual. This classification is explained in ancient nādi texts and we are now learning this in the twenty-first century. These ancient texts tried to bridge subjectivity and objectivity.

To learn this technique, go to the deepest pulse at the seventh level. Then gently release the pressure and come to the sixth level, where the spike changes. At the seventh level, the spike will be felt at the center of the lotus. With a slight release of pressure to the sixth level, the direction of the pulse under each finger will be felt towards one of the petals of the lotus. Try to focus attention under each finger separately. Under the vāta finger find out whether the spike is at the Indra, Agni, Yama, or other position. Take a note of the reading. Then turn your attention to the pitta finger and find the direction of the spike, and then feel the kapha finger and do the same. The tip of the finger is held perpendicular to the radial artery and you feel the middle of the artery. The spike usually moves in the direction of one petal, but it may even move to more than one petal or stay at the center.

With this information, the person's manas prakruti can be understood as a mixed prakruti of deity characteristics and vāta, pitta and kapha. The spike under each finger is likely to be at different petals of the lotus. We are all a mixture of the three doshas and three gunas and every person generally has a manas prakruti with the characteristics of three of the deities. The qualities of each deity merge with those of the related dosha, which helps us to clarify our understanding of the individual's personality. The strongest spike indicates the most prominent deity. For example, if someone has spikes of Indra, Varuna and Kubera, they will have characteristics of all three deities. However, the strongest spike of these three shows which is the ruling deity in that prakruti. Don't compare the reading with the prakruti of the subject; instead just feel the direction of the spike while visualizing the lotus.

Manas prakruti can also be studied directly using the three gunas: sattva, rajas and tamas. In that scheme, we can feel for spikes in the same positions on each finger as are used for the prakruti and vikruti pulses. A spike in the vāta or distal position of any finger indicates rajas, while a spike at the central curvature in the pitta position shows sattva, and one in the kapha or proximal site represents tamas guna. However, that results in a broad classification that can be too limiting. The eight-petaled flower under each finger gives a more appropriate description of the person's manas prakruti (and manas vikruti), so that the personality of each deity can be applied to the readings on the sixth and second levels.

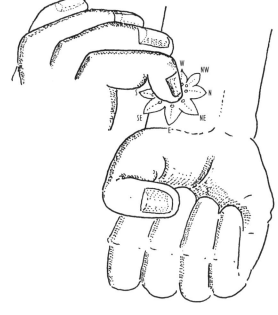

Firstly read your own manas prakruti and then try to feel others' manas prakruti pulse. In regards to the illustration of the hand and petals, the fingertips of the person being examined are visualized as pointing to the east. Therefore, it is ideal for the subject to face east and the reader to face west, to simplify the reading. Keep stationary the finger reading the pulse. Use the right hand of the person for a man and the left hand for a woman. The lotus is in the same position on both hands, so don't become confused by the position of the subject's thumb in the illustration.

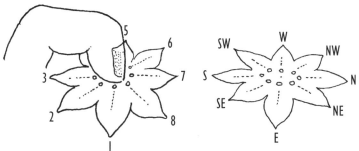

One can read an eight-petaled lotus under all three of the fingers, but that is too complicated initially. For beginners, it is better to use only the finger with the most prominent spike. For example, if it is under the index finger, read the manas prakruti under this finger, because the mind and consciousness are expressing strongest through that spike of the pulse. Suppose throbbing is felt relatively strongly under two fingers, such as the index and middle fingers. Compare which is more prominent and visualize the eight-petaled lotus under that finger. This is imagination, but the greatest scientist is gifted with the positive power of imagination. Be a scientist and be imaginative.

PLANETARY PRINCIPLES IN THE NĀDI

The sixth level of the pulse can also denote planetary principles acting in the nādi, although these readings may not correspond to one's *Jyotish* astrological birth chart. The sixth level of the pulse indicates the status of the mental body. The modern term astral body is composed of the ancient Upanishad descriptions of the prāna body and the manas body. The movement of prāna becomes disturbed by the vibrations of thoughts, feelings and emotions coming from the manas body. So the mental body can affect the prāna body, and the prāna body can disturb the mental body. Before pathological changes happen in the physical body, subtle changes take place in the mental and prāna bodies. In other words, the astral body plays an indirect role in the immune system, affecting agni, tejas and ojas.

Many times people ask what gemstone they should wear, on which day they should fast, or which deity they should worship. The sixth level of the pulse reveals this information. Read each finger in the same way as for manas prakruti. For example, if the reading of the petals denotes $V_2P_3K_7$, the table below shows that 2 on the vāta finger represents the Moon, so the person should wear a pearl. Petal Number 3 on the pitta finger is Mars, indicating the person should wear red coral. Hence with this combination of vāta and pitta, the person should wear a red coral necklace with a pearl in the center. Petal Number 7 on the kapha finger represents Jupiter and the stone to be used is a yellow sapphire. Using the correct gems facilitates healing. The relationships between planets, gemstones, deities and fasting days are shown in the table below, while the whole of the next chapter is devoted to the qualities and actions of some commonly used gemstones.

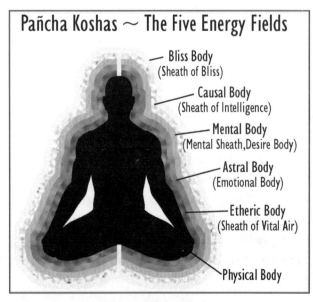

Pañcha Koshas ~ The Five Energy Fields

— Bliss Body
(Sheath of Bliss)

— Causal Body
(Sheath of Intelligence)

— Mental Body
(Mental Sheath, Desire Body)

— Astral Body
(Emotional Body)

— Etheric Body
(Sheath of Vital Air)

— Physical Body

Life without a personal deity is without direction, leading to a feeling of ungroundedness. When anchored with a deity, one will never feel lonely or ungrounded. One's connection with a personal deity brings stability, direction and perfume to life. Then the whole life becomes celebration, not a meaningless futile game. It is difficult to have a direct relationship with Almighty God, but worship of a personal deity such as Ganesha, Vishnu, Rāma, Krishna, Christ or Buddha brings communion with higher consciousness. Almighty God is experienced through the personal deity and this deity becomes a bridge to salvation and enlightenment. The table on page 112 is a guide in the choice of the right gemstone and deity.

The choice is also guided by which doshas are active in the manas prakruti and vikruti. For instance, if vāta is active, the person could wear a moonstone, which is a stone that will calm vāta. There is a bridge between dosha, planets and gemstones in manas prakruti. When one fasts on a specified day, the blessing of that particular planet is received. In Āyurveda, there is a branch of astrology called astrotherapy (*graha chikitsā*), which addresses the influences of the planets upon the person.

Suppose a person has a pitta problem and under the pitta finger the spike is in the Mars position (Petal Number 3). The high pitta is due to the affliction of Mars in the mind. Wearing a red coral necklace will absorb the Mars energy, while fasting on Tuesday will calm down pitta and the Mars-provoking influence. Fasting according to these principles will eliminate mental impurities or āma.

Enlightenment has many doors and there are many paths to realization. God never asks through which door you come, in which car you arrive or on which flight. He is just happy to see you and bless you. There are many ways to become enlightened—*mantra yoga, jñāna yoga, bhakti yoga, karma yoga,* chanting the holy name of God, fasting, doing *pūjā,* doing worship—all these ways lead to God. Therefore, one's entire life becomes a celebration.

Planetary Influences in the Nādi

ﻉ Vāta
△ Pitta
▢ Kapha

1) Venus - Diamond
2) Moon - Pearl
3) Mars - Red coral
4) Rahu - Gomed
5) Saturn - Blue Sapphire
6) Ketu - Moonstone
7) Jupiter - Yellow Sapphire
8) Mercury - Emerald
9) Sun - Ruby

Āyurvedic culture makes life a ceremony. Even death becomes a ceremony. People take the body, carry it to the cremation yard, chant mantra, burn the body to ashes and carry the ashes to the sacred river. The deceased person's soul is happy and that soul has equal energy to that of God. Therefore, never speak bad things about a deceased person. This is very important. A person makes his life miserable if he carries unresolved emotions about a deceased father or mother. Never ever carry unresolved anger about a deceased person. When a person has ceased to exist physically, that anger should be resolved and released.

Table 8: Planets and Deities

PLANET	GEMSTONE	FASTING DAY	DEITY
Sun (Center)	Ruby (mānikyam)	Sunday	Rāma; Gayatrī Devī; Christ
Venus (Petal #1)	Diamond (vajra)	Friday	Lakshmī; Sarasvatī; Durga; Allah; Balaji
Moon (Petal #2)	Pearl (moti)	Monday	Shiva
Mars (Petal #3)	Red coral (pravāla)	Tuesday	Ganesha
Rāhu (Petal #4)	Gomed (tapomani)	Monday	Rāhu
Saturn (Petal #5)	Blue Sapphire (nīlam)	Saturday	Shani Deva; Hanuman
Ketu (Petal #6)	Moonstone (vaidūrya, lasnya)	Thursday	Ketu
Jupiter (Petal #7)	Yellow Sapphire (pushkarāja)	Thursday	Dattatraya; Lakshmī
Mercury (Petal #8)	Emerald (harinmani)	Wednesday	Vithala; Vishnu; Krishna; Buddha

The deities related to the Sun are Rāma, Gayatrī Devī and Christ. Shiva is related to the Moon and Monday is a good day to worship Shiva. Mars is connected to Lord Ganesha and, when Mars is activated, Ganesha will cool down that Mars energy. Mercury is related to Lord Vithala, Krishna and Vishnu, as well as Buddha. Jupiter relates to Lord Dattatraya and Lakshmī. Venus, which is connected to Friday, is worshipped through Lakshmī, Sarasvatī, Durga, Balaji and Allah. Saturday is Lord Shani and Hanuman. Hanuman is also worshipped to calm down Mars. According to Vedic philosophy, Hanuman is a living entity who is the son of the Wind God and travels with the speed of the wind. He is the dedicated servant of Rāma. Hanuman is full of love. He stands for bhakti and service. He protects us from evil energy, such as ghosts and spirits. Chanting the *Hanuman Chalisa* on Saturday and Tuesday will activate this protective energy. Rāhu and Ketu are pleased by worshipping them on Saturday and Tuesday respectively. Fasting from sunrise to sunset is a good discipline, cleansing the body, mind and consciousness. For fasting, take fruits or fruit juice, which are sattvic, and don't eat any cooked grains.

In the Hindu religion there are about 36,000 deities. The Hindus worship everything as a manifestation of God—trees, flowers, and there is even a special day for cows. They also worship the bull, which is a vehicle of Lord Shiva. They are innocent like a child and innocence is the perfume of life. Knowledge is beautiful but knowledge makes the person rigid and logical. Logic is based upon knowledge and reasoning. On the other hand, intelligence is creative. Hence, logic has no intelligence.

CHAKRAS IN THE PULSE

The word chakra means wheel and chakras are centers of energy in the body related to physical, mental and spiritual energies. If the flow of energy in any of these centers becomes blocked, stress is reflected in the physiology. The sixth level of the pulse reveals how well each of these chakras is functioning. Reading this information is slightly different from determining the manas prakruti.

The pulse felt by the ring finger at the proximal curvature denotes the activity of *mūlādhāra*, the first chakra. The activity of *svādhisthāna*, the second chakra, is felt at the distal curvature of the same finger. On the middle finger, one can detect *manipūra* (third) and *anāhata* (fourth) chakras at the proximal and distal positions, respectively.

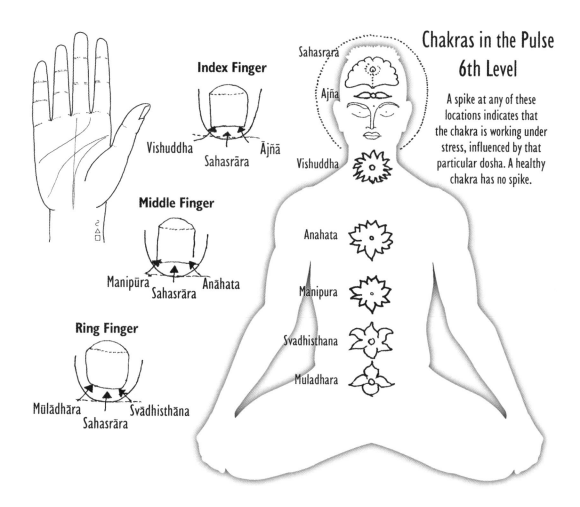

Chakras in the Pulse
6th Level

A spike at any of these locations indicates that the chakra is working under stress, influenced by that particular dosha. A healthy chakra has no spike.

On the index finger, one will feel *vishuddha* (fifth) and *ājñā* (sixth) chakras. The central part of each finger denotes the activity of sahasrāra. When a spike is present, it indicates that chakra is working under stress and the kundalinī shakti is blocked there. That chakra needs cleansing work. A healthy chakra has no spike, showing the *kundalinī* energy is moving smoothly. A dynamo that works perfectly creates no noise, whereas a dynamo that is cracked creates a loud noise. Similarly, a chakra that is working under stress creates a spike.

We are ordinary people who are involved with worldly affairs, so our chakras may not be open. What is the spike of an enlightened person? An enlightened person will have a gentle, balanced spike at the site of sahasrāra that expands like a lotus under all three fingers.

The *bīja mantra* for each chakra is given below. '*Lam*' is for mūlādhāra, '*vam*' for svādhisthāna, '*ram*' for manipūra, '*yam*' for anāhata, '*ham*' for vishuddha, '*sham-ksham*' for ājñā, and '*so-hum*' for sahasrāra. The mantra '*aum*' is for bliss, and its effects are located about the width of 10 fingers above the physical brain, which is the junction between the auric field and cosmic consciousness. This point is called *anuchāra*, which means the unspoken soundless sound, the sound of one hand clapping. It is a sound without duality. If the person mentally recites the appropriate mantra 108 times, that helps to release the blockage and open the chakra. The chakra system and chromo-therapy go together. The seven rainbow colors are red, orange, yellow, green, blue, indigo and violet, and they are also the colors of the chakras, from mūlādhāra to sahasrāra respectively.

A spike at mūlādhāra on the proximal curvature of the ring finger may be connected to the reproductive organs—testicles, ovaries, cervix and prostate. The person may have sexual debility or low libido. If the spike is on the distal curvature of the ring finger, it is connected to the second chakra, svādhisthāna—kidney, urethra, bladder and adrenals. The second chakra is also connected to the spleen and gov-

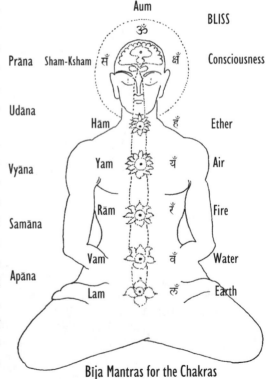

Bija Mantras for the Chakras

erns the water element. The third chakra is functionally connected to the stomach, pancreas, small intestine, liver and gallbladder. The fourth chakra relates to the heart and lungs and the fifth to the vocal cords, thyroid and parathyroid. The sixth is related to the third eye and the pituitary gland and the seventh to the pineal gland.

With this understanding, now try to read your own chakra pulse, and then read the condition of your friend's chakra pulse. Again, the right hand in the man and the left hand in the woman should be used to understand the chakras. To find this pulse at the sixth level, gently tune your finger to locate the presence of the spike. Try to contact the throb. This information is at the same sixth level as manas prakruti and the planetary influences, but the fine tuning is different. A spike at sahasrāra on the kapha finger means the crown chakra has a tarpaka kapha disorder. A spike at sahasrāra under the pitta finger indicates sādhaka pitta is involved. If a sahasrāra spike is under the index finger, prāna vāta is involved. An uneven spike at the sahasrāra site under all three fingers means the person is mentally disturbed. But if the spikes are equally balanced at this position under all three fingers, the person is enlightened.

THE PRESENT FLOW OF CONSCIOUSNESS

Now we will shift our attention to the second level. Just a bit below the superficial pulse on the first level, the spike changes. The second level represents the present flow of consciousness. Although we refer to this present flow of consciousness as manas vikruti, it is more appropriately called the present status of the mind. Under each finger visualize the eight-petaled lotus representing the eight directions, in the same manner as at the sixth level. This pulse changes approximately every 90 minutes, due to changing thought waves and feelings. It is not permanent, because it is a flow of consciousness connected to the thought waves. At one moment there may be a wave of sadness and depression; at the next moment, one may feel happy.

A spike in the east direction (Petal Number 1) represents creative, positive thoughts. A spike in the southeast (Petal Number 2) represents judgmental thoughts, which sometimes manifest as self-criticism or perfectionism. Pitta people are often perfectionistic, which creates stress in them. A spike in the south (Petal Number 3) indicates grief, sadness, depression and loneliness. The fourth direction is southwest (Petal Number 4), representing pessimistic thinking, worthlessness and depression. The west direction (Petal Number 5) is related to passion, attachment and emotional thinking. Attachment can be to anything. People are attached to status, relationships and objects. The northwest direction (Petal Number 6) represents emotional thinking and a chattering mind, and north (Petal Number 7) indicates thinking of money and success. Northeast (Petal Number 8) is spiritual thought and the mind is calm, quiet and serene. If all three fingers have a spike at the center, it indicates a quiet mind that is in meditation. Such a pulse indicates that the person is at one with the present.

This level may or may not be the same as the manas prakruti at the sixth level. For example, a person may be born with a sattvic manas prakruti, with a spike at Ishanya, but may become predominantly rajasic in his or her manas vikruti as he or she reaches adulthood, with a spike felt at petal number two.

An important aspect of Indian philosophy is the theory of the five elements, which is closely linked to the three doshas. Each of the celestial elements has a representative form—a circle for Space; hexagon for Air; triangle, Fire; crescent, Water; square, Earth. The same principle is applied to the hand. The thumb represents Space, the index finger is Air, the middle finger is Fire, ring finger is Water, and the little finger is Earth. As we explained in Chapter One, one can get the client to breathe onto a mirror and observe the shape formed by the person's exhaled breath. This relates to the shapes of the elements, which influence the body and the mind, and it will give us an indication of the most prominent element at that moment of time. This test can be used to confirm the findings of the second level pulse, as related to the elements for each petal that are shown in the table.

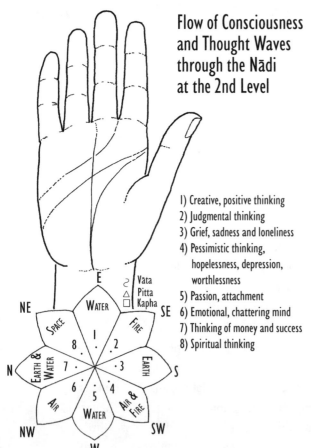

Flow of Consciousness and Thought Waves through the Nādi at the 2nd Level

1) Creative, positive thinking
2) Judgmental thinking
3) Grief, sadness and loneliness
4) Pessimistic thinking, hopelessness, depression, worthlessness
5) Passion, attachment
6) Emotional, chattering mind
7) Thinking of money and success
8) Spiritual thinking

Now we will try to read the second level of the pulse. First read your own pulse, and then your friend's second level pulse. Keep the fingers still. For comparison, use each finger separately. Perhaps the vāta finger may indicate depression but the pitta finger may show judgmental thinking and the kapha finger a spiritual attribute. That which is overpowering will rule your present flow of consciousness. Feel under each finger and then we will learn to interpret. Read the pulse on the right hand for the male and the left hand for the female. Remember that this pulse reveals what the person is thinking at the present moment.

Creative thoughts are sattvic and judgmental thoughts are rajasic, and rajasic people like to compare. Depressive thoughts are tamasic. Grief and sadness can be either rajasic or tamasic. Chattering is rajasic, thinking of money is rajasic and spiritual thinking is sattvic. These three qualities—sattva, rajas and tamas—flow through the superficial pulse at the second level.

As with the previous pulses in this chapter, the fingers of the person being examined are always visualized as facing east and it is the direction of the spike that determines the number of the petal. This present flow of consciousness changes according to the person's situation, responsibility and events that occur in one's life. The superficial pulse at the second level is connected moment-to-moment with our thought waves, and thought is a biochemical vehicle through which we communicate with the throb of the pulse. If this second level is checked in the morning, afternoon and evening, changes will be noticed.

Vāta, pitta and kapha have different significance at this level of the pulse. Vāta, when being creative and positive, comes like a breeze and goes away. It is a temporary phase. Pitta, when creative and positive, is a deep and concentrated state of being. Kapha, when creative and positive, lasts a long time, because kapha moves slowly. Consider every aspect of the dosha. Pitta is judgmental. Vāta is also judgmental, but the judgmental quality of vāta is not that deep. It will be here for a while and then go away. Whereas when pitta people judge, they judge.

It is important to pay attention to the breath while examining the subject. Watch the movement of the person's chest. When the person is breathing in, you should be breathing out, as if you are putting your apāna in the person's prāna. Conversely, you also take that person's apāna into your prāna with your inhalation. However, you should exercise caution with this practice, because you may receive the energies of the subject and pick up the person's feelings and emotions. To feel someone's pulse is an energy exchange. There are certain methods to protect one's self. Practice So-Hum meditation and watch the breath. In addition, wearing gemstones and crystals such as amethyst, rose quartz and a rudraksha *mālā* will add protection. One can also practice the meditation of passive awareness, during which there is doing without the sense of the doer.

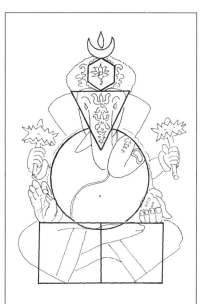

Ganesha is an elephant-headed God in Hindu mythology. His embodiment represents an expression of the five universal elements. They are as follows:

The crossed legs, represented by a square, are a manifestation of the physical world through the Earth element.

His belly, shown by a circle, depicts the Space element, which is a vast universal womb, pregnant with billions of galaxies.

His face, denoted by a triangle, is a symbol of the Fire element, which expresses cosmic wisdom.

The hexagonal crown is a symbol of the Air element, which denotes cosmic prāna, the flow of intelligence.

The crescent over the crown is a symbol of soma, the pure essence of cosmic Water. It also represents the mastery over the cosmic mind at the time of creation.

On the top of the crescent is a flame of light, which is the flame of pure awareness and bliss.

Emotions can enter through the breath. When one unconsciously breathes in, one can take in another person's energy. Even when walking by someone on the street who is throwing out thoughts of anger and fear, these molecules and atoms of thoughts can be inhaled. When arriving home, feelings of sadness come up without any apparent reason. We have picked up that person's energy. Conscious breathing and the So-Hum mantra are important. When practicing So-Hum meditation, one does not incorporate other people's energy. One remains alert and tranquil.

There are many ways to improve the sensitivity in the fingers. One is to rub the fingers with certain medicated oils containing brahmi and vacha, which bring more alertness and sensitive observation. I always do So-Hum meditation when I feel the pulse. With So-Hum, the mind, thoughts and feelings do not interfere, and the perception of the pulse becomes clear. Or use any guru-given authentic mantra. A mantra can neutralize the blockage and interference created by one's own thoughts and pulsations. Examining an individual's pulse is meditation. Meditate, feel the pulse, focus attention on the mantra and the pulse will be present under your fingers. In this way the reading will be accurate.

Practically, the sixth level of manas prakruti doesn't usually change unless one becomes enlightened. When one transcends normal consciousness, that person is beyond manas prakruti. To practice meditation is to go beyond manas prakruti. Up to this point, pulse reading has been more technical, but to realize the subtleties of the pulse needs sensitive awareness. The concepts presented in this chapter are complicated and will bring up many questions in the mind of the reader. However, all these questions can be answered by the development of subjective perception.

Specific Conditions of Manas Vikruti
Certain conditions of manas vikruti can be assessed from the pulse as a whole, rather than using the second level only. The following are two examples.

Unmāda (Mania or Psychosis). Check at all levels for the feeling of the pulse as a whole. If, in all the levels, there is a strong pitta spike under the index finger, a slow, deep, wavy kapha quality under the middle finger, and fast, feeble vāta pulsations under the ring finger, as shown in the diagram, the pulse reveals unmāda (psychosis) or a form of mania.

Bhūtonmāda (Psychosis Due to Influence of an Evil Spirit). Characteristics of this pulse are similar to those felt in the unmāda pulse—a pitta spike under the index finger, a kapha spike under the middle finger and a vāta spike beneath the ring finger. However, the pulse will be imbedded deep within the flesh. This condition is indicative of a form of mania due to possession.

In other cases, the person has a staring look and a shadowed personality and the pulse is small and thready under all three fingers. It is cold to the touch and shows extreme vāta. We are not talking about a particular level of the pulse here. This kind of pulse is beyond the levels and it is present when a person is influenced by an evil spirit. The pulse in general can be masked by the prakruti of the spirit. The spirit is a localized energy field that moves like a wave or a breeze, passing through the person's auric field. First the aura is clouded, then the mind is disturbed, and finally the body can be affected. In this condition, there is a total change in personality and behavior from one's normal behavior. When the person's appearance suggests one dosha as predominant in the prakruti but the pulse shows another dosha, this indicates possession. We can't prove this objectively, but we can see that the person's behavior pattern is quite different. This pulse becomes prominent during the full moon and new moon, when conditions such as schizophrenia, double personality and psychosis are more active. The person can be treated by giving management primarily for vāta dosha.

THE EFFECTS OF GEMSTONES AND CRYSTALS ON THE PULSE

Gemstones and crystals can have subtle influences on vāta, pitta and kapha. The healing energy of these stones can be activated in the individual by wearing them as ornaments such as rings or necklaces, or by placing them in water overnight and drinking the water the next day. Gems give off and draw in energy through their negative and positive vibrations. They should, therefore, be purified, such as by placing them in salt water for two days. Gemstones activate the energy centers in the body and in this way help to develop sensitivity.

The healers in ancient Vedic times studied gemology by observing the subtle effects of gemstones on the doshas and actions on the pulse. As we have seen, there are many pulses in the body—seven levels and three fingers makes 21 pulses on the right side and another 21 on the left. For convenience, if we only study the superficial and deep levels, including the pulses of the organs, we will gain much information. That knowledge is enough for beginning the study of the effects of gems and crystals on the pulse.

Understanding how planets and deities and their related gemstones are prescribed is important. The gemstone or crystal should touch the skin through a little window in the setting, so that the subtle energies of the stone can interact more directly with the energies of the body. Generally, a gemstone is worn as a ring. A pearl (Moon) or emerald (Mercury) should be worn on the little finger, a ruby (Sun), diamond (Venus) or red coral (Mars) on the ring finger, yellow sapphire (Jupiter) on the index finger, and blue sapphire (Saturn) is the only gem to be worn on the middle finger. Gomed (Rāhu) can go on either the ring or little finger, and moonstone (Ketu) on the little finger. There is no ring for the thumb, because the thumb represents the soul (*angustha purusha*). In general, gems that are heating should be set in silver, but there are some exceptions.

The "day" of a gemstone is based on the related deity. It is considered important for setting the stone and first wearing it. Just as in marriage, when two elements come together and yield something new, a gem and its mount yield a new sphere of influence—as a ring and a medicine. It is considered auspicious to unite these on the day of the deity to be honored and pacified. Further, donning the ring for the first time on this day is important for the same reason. The vibration of the gem works best along certain pathways of energy (nādis). Therefore, gems and their energies are matched with specific nādis, which affect physiology in known ways.

Some diamonds and other gems carry a curse. Although it is fashionable now to buy antique jewelry, we do not know who previously wore it. The energy of the person remains with the jewelry and needs to be cleared before a new person wears it.

Processed or chemically treated stones may not have the same healing energy. It is best to get authentic, unprocessed, clean stones, without any flaw or crack. Never wear a cracked stone. The cutting of the gemstone should be even and symmetrical. When buying a stone, use a magnifying glass or microscope to examine its quality. The size of most stones should be three to five carats, although a one carat diamond is large enough.

A gemstone or crystal can also be taken internally in the form of a *bhasma* or alchemic ash, specially prepared by Āyurvedic methods. This gives prompt and accurate results. Every gemstone has *rasa* (taste), *vīrya* (heating or cooling energy) and *vipāka* (post-digestive effects). However these can only be clearly observed in the body if the bhasma is taken internally. The taste is not evident if one just licks the gem. Wearing gemstones and crystals as rings or necklaces has a more subtle effect on the auric field, but the rasa, vīrya and vipāka will all have an effect on the doshas.

Ruby (padmarāga mani or mānikyam)

Astrologically, the ruby represents the sun. The ruby is a precious stone, sweet and pungent to the taste, heating and with a sweet post-digestive effect. The external use of ruby, either in the form of a necklace or a ring worn on the ring finger, has a subtle effect on the pulse and doshas. Ruby pacifies vāta and kapha but may elevate pitta. If a pitta person puts on a ruby, the pulse may become high, jumping and bounding like a frog. This pitta aggravation can ultimately cause hives, rash and acne. Garnet and ruby have the same vibration and garnet is a poor man's ruby. Ruby is a life-giving stone and gives increased longevity to vāta and kapha people. It brings prosperity and kindles agni, improving digestion. If a vāta or kapha person is sick, ruby may help to heal, calming the vāta and kapha spikes to a normal level.

Pearl (moti)

Pearl is called moti. There is an interesting story about the pearl. Pearls are found in the mother shell because sand enters and creates an irritation, causing the oozing of a mucous secretion that eventually covers the sand forming a pearl. However that is an ordinary pearl. On a full moon day during the period of *svāti nakshatra* (a special star), a white cloud appears when the moon is rising. When that particular cloud starts raining on the ocean, a Mother Pearl comes to the surface, opens her mouth and swallows one drop of that water. On the full moon, that drop of water from the cloud carries the quality and nectar of the moon, and that moon sweat is swallowed by the Mother Pearl. She meditates upon that drop. It takes a minimum of six months and a maximum of one-and-a-half years to transform that drop of water into a pearl. This is a special pearl, which has a slight bluish-white color.

Pearl is sweet, cooling and has a sweet post-digestive effect. Pearl balances all three doshas. Astrologically, pearl is a symbol of the moon. In Āyurveda, pearl bhasma is used for gastritis, gastric ulcer, peptic ulcer and sexual debility. Used externally, it is effective when any of the three doshas is high. Pearl is good for everyone, because it brings mental peace and tranquility. In particular, pearl brings a high pitta spike back to normal. For those with pitta as the predominant dosha, a pearl should be set in silver. For kapha and vāta doshas, gold is the preferred setting. It should be worn on the little finger or, in some special conditions, on the index finger. Consult your Vedic astrologer.

Gomed (tapomani)

Gomed is sour to the taste, has a heating vīrya, and the post-digestive effect is pungent. It pacifies vāta and kapha but stimulates pitta. It has a direct action on rakta and māmsa dhātus. Gomed improves the digestion and strengthens the solar plexus and spleen. Whenever the spleen pulse is feeble or if a person has muscle fatigue, gomed can be useful. It is also helpful in attention deficit disorder. Gomed should be worn on the ring finger and set in gold.

Yellow Sapphire (pushkarāja)

Pushkarāja is sweet, cooling, and the post-digestive effect is sweet. It calms vāta and pitta, but may slightly build kapha. Pushkarāja represents Jupiter and brings groundedness and stability. When a person has a vāta or pitta disorder with ungroundedness and instability, a yellow sapphire or topaz in a gold setting on the right index finger helps the person become more stable. Yellow sapphire should go with gold, but from the Jyotish point of view, it can sometimes be put in copper or silver to calm down the negative effects of Mars or the Moon. It should always be worn on the index finger, which is the finger of Guru, Jupiter.

When meda and majjā dhātu pulses are prominent, pushkarāja brings balance. In addition, it is beneficial when a person has atrial flutter with fibrillation. It also strengthens the heart and builds kidney and lung energy. Yellow sapphire is more expensive than topaz, which is the poor man's sapphire. However, yellow topaz can be used as a substitute, as it has the same rasa, vīrya and vipāka as yellow sapphire.

Red Coral (pravāla)
Red coral is called pravāla. It is sweet and pungent, cooling, and the post-digestive effect is sweet. It is tridoshic. Coral bhasma cools down pitta and it is effectively used when the pulse shows low liver, spleen and pericardial energy. Coral particularly gives energy to the liver and it protects from Mars energy. Astrologically, an affliction of Mars can produce pitta disorders and liver problems. Wearing a red coral necklace or a ring set in copper and worn on the ring finger will protect the liver, spleen and pericardium. Some people do not tolerate copper. In that case, silver or white gold is equally good. In Āyurveda coral bhasma is used internally to heal gastric ulcer and cholecystitis.

Diamond (vajra)
Vajra is a variety of diamond that is difficult to break. Only another diamond can break a diamond. Vajra is pungent and astringent, heating with a pungent post-digestive effect. Vajra calms all three doshas, but some pitta people may not tolerate diamond very well. A vajra diamond prevents premature aging, enhances the span of life and strengthens immunity. In addition, it stimulates sexual energy, because a diamond represents Venus, which governs the reproductive system. Art, music, romance and sex all go together with this stone. A diamond should be set in gold and can be worn as a necklace or as a ring on the ring finger.

Blue Sapphire (nīlam)
Blue sapphire is called nīlam and it is pungent, heating, and its post-digestive effect is pungent. The blue sapphire represents Saturn and it calms vāta and kapha, but stimulates pitta. When Saturn is active in a person's horoscope, the musculo-skeletal system may be affected. Blue sapphire acts on māmsa dhātu (the muscle tissue) and asthi dhātu (the bones). It prevents emaciation and protects from an affliction of Saturn, and one will receive the benefits of Saturn while wearing this stone. Saturn, a deity of earth and the metal iron, is a spiritual planet that represents renunciation, austerity and harsh discipline, and it brings transcendental experiences and enlightenment. Saturn shows every person his or her right place, but it may bring loneliness and depression. The vehicle of

Saturn is hamsa, the swan, which is also the vehicle of Sarasvatī and Brahma, the Creator.

Blue sapphire is the only stone worn on the right middle finger and it is better to place it in a silver setting. It helps to build up the muscles and skeletal system and it can heal arthritic changes. When the pulse is feeble and vāta is high, use blue sapphire. Never wear a diamond and blue sapphire together on the same finger. This will suppress the person's sexual energy and create disharmony in a relationship.

Lapis Lazuli (indranīla)
Lapis lazuli is bitter, has a cooling vīrya, and the post-digestive effect is sweet. It calms vāta and pitta and may build kapha. This gem regulates bile and is a blood cleanser. Lapis lazuli is good for skin diseases and bleeding disorders. Use indranīla when a person has anxiety, fear and weakness in the heart. It should be set in gold and can be worn on the little finger.

Emerald (harinmani)
Emerald is sweet, cooling, and has a sweet post-digestive effect. It calms vāta and pitta, but may stimulate kapha. This stone is cooling but, because of its *prabhāva*, it calms the nervous system and improves the power of speech. It is nutritive, digestive, and brings prosperity and spiritual awakening. Emerald is worn on the little finger and should be set in gold.

Moonstone (vaidūrya, lasnya)
Lasnya is pungent, heating, and the post-digestive effect is pungent. It calms vāta and kapha, but it may slightly stimulate pitta dosha. This stone is good for allergies, repeated colds and congestion, and asthma. It also aids in healing kidney dysfunction. Moonstone enhances awareness, so a person doesn't get caught in his or her emotions. People working in psychological healing should wear lasnya in a gold setting on the little or ring finger to protect them from negative vibrations. This stone also protects from evil spirits.

Sūryākānta
Sūryākānta is a very special stone. It is pink in color and looks like rose quartz. If held in the sunlight, it oozes water and starts sweating. This stone acts on māmsa and majjā dhātus. It is sweet, heating, and the post-digestive effect is sweet. It pacifies vāta, may stimulate pitta and calms kapha. It also improves memory. When a person has a tendency toward seizures and poor memory, sūryākānta helps. It should be set in gold and worn on the ring finger.

Quartz Crystal (sphatika)

Quartz crystals are pungent and sweet, cooling and have a sweet post-digestive effect. They calm vāta, but because of the pungent taste, some pitta people do not tolerate quartz crystal. The sweet taste and vipāka and cooling energy of quartz also stimulates kapha. Quartz crystals attract radioactive energy. They are good for fistulae and prickly heat, and they improve the quality of perception. They also enhance intuition. Quartz crystals can be set in either silver or gold and worn as a necklace or as a ring on the ring finger. When the pericardial pulse is feeble, quartz crystals may help to strengthen that pulse.

Onyx (tribhuja, harita pīta mani)

Onyx is pungent, heating and the post-digestive effect is pungent. It calms vāta and kapha, but may aggravate pitta. Onyx is good for old age, debilitating disorders and neurological dysfunctions. It works on the rakta, māmsa and majjā dhātus. Onyx induces quiet sleep and improves the power of sleep. It is also good for memory, positive thinking and lethargy, and it is a good gem for tarpaka kapha. Onyx makes life peaceful and happy, and it enhances love in a relationship. If one wears onyx, evil spirits will not come near. This stone should be set in silver and worn on the ring finger. Astrologically, if the Sun sign is in Sagittarius or Gemini in a Vedic astrology chart, one should not wear this stone.

Bloodstone (lohita, jyotirāja)

Bloodstone is sour and pungent, heating, and the post-digestive effect is pungent. It is warming and is a good blood cleanser. It stimulates pitta, but calms both vāta and kapha. Bloodstone gives energy and warmth, improves circulation, and builds the liver and gallbladder energies. It can be set in either silver or copper and should be worn on the little finger.

Jade (nephrite, yashava, bhisma pashan)

Jade is sour and pungent, slightly heating and the vipāka is pungent. It calms vāta and kapha and it stimulates pitta. This stone strengthens kidney energy and is reputed to bestow success upon its wearer. If the kidney pulse is low and the person has a tendency to form kidney stones, jade is good to protect the kidneys from various maladies. It also increases longevity and the power of speech, it prevents cataracts and abdominal pain, and provides protection from black magic. Jade should be set in silver and worn on the little finger.

Amethyst (nīla sphatika)

Amethyst can be purple, pinkish or indigo in color. It is sweet and cooling and its post-digestive effect is sweet. It is balancing to all three doshas, although excessive exposure can stimulate vāta. Amethyst is a stone for the crown chakra and is good for mental clarity. It acts on majjā dhātu. Amethyst is best set in gold, to bring prosperity. Some amethysts have a darker color, which gives them a sapphire-like energy. A person with neuromuscular weakness can be helped by wearing amethyst and by putting amethyst crystals at the four corners of the bed to protect the auric field. Amethyst will provide protection from electromagnetic energy and radiation and can be used to protect the corners of one's house from negative energy.

Opal (sāgararāja, varuna)

Opal is a semi-precious stone with sweet taste and cooling energy. It has a sweet post-digestive effect. Opal can increase vāta and kapha and it calms pitta dosha. Opal represents the planet Neptune. It has black, white, bluish or gentle green shades of color and it is soft and brittle. Opal acts on majjā and shukra dhātus and it increases the strength of these dhātu pulses. It aids in improving vision and relieves fever. By its prabhāva, it unfolds spiritual feelings, bhakti (devotion) and intuition. When this gem looks bright, something "good" will happen. If the stone looks dull and shadowed, something unpleasant will happen in the near future. Opal is good for people with Pisces as a rising sign. When the planet Neptune is in the third, fourth, sixth, eighth, tenth or twelfth house, this gem is quite beneficial. It should be set in gold or silver and worn on the ring finger.

Alexandrite (hemaratna, harshal)

Alexandrite changes its color due to changes in the reflection of the sun. In the morning, it looks greenish-purple, during midday it appears reddish-indigo, and in the evening it shows a greenish-red color. Because of this quality of changing color, Alexandrite is considered to be a precious gem. It is sweet and sour to the taste, with cooling vīrya and a sweet post-digestive effect. It aggravates vāta and kapha and pacifies pitta. Alexandrite brings tranquillity to the mind and affects the nervous system and the majjā dhātu pulse. It enhances memory and is also beneficial for a person with grand mal epilepsy. This gem brings good luck. It should be set in gold and worn on the ring finger.

Aquamarine (harita nīla mani)

The color of aquamarine is sky blue or greenish-blue, and it looks like sea water. Aquamarine is also called "Sea Green." Its taste is sweet and astringent, with cooling vīrya and a post-digestive effect of sweet. It is balancing to all three doshas. Aquamarine acts on rakta, māmsa and shukra dhātus and it strengthens these dhātu pulses. It eliminates dullness of the mind and brings mental happiness and intelligence. Aquamarine also promotes the power of speech and memory. It is good for married couples to wear this stone to enhance love in their relationship. Aquamarine is a substitute for emerald. It should be set in silver and worn on the little finger.

The element of faith is important when connected with wearing these gemstones. Faith moves the mountain. If one has faith and trust in the person giving the stone, it will work as a healing factor. So the effect of these gems does have a connection to faith. Modern medicine considers faith a placebo effect, but Āyurveda says that faith is more than a placebo. It has a direct connection with spirit, consciousness and innermost awareness.

Table 9: Gemstones and Their Effects

GEMSTONE	EFFECT	PLANET
Ruby (padmarāga mani or mānikyam)	Sweet and pungent, heating, sweet. Regulates action of vāta and kapha but may stimulate pitta. Promotes long life. Good for poor circulation, anemia and spleen dysfunctions.	Sun
Pearl (moti)	Sweet, cooling, sweet. Tridoshic. Calms the mind. Nutritious and strengthening for rasa, māmsa and shukra dhātus.	Moon
Gomed (tapomani)	Sour, heating, pungent. Pacifies vāta and kapha, stimulates pitta. Improves digestion and circulation. Strengthens solar plexus and spleen. Helps lymphatic congestion and edema. Good for attention deficit disorder.	Rāhu
Yellow Sapphire (pushkarāja)	Sweet, cooling, sweet. Regulates vāta, calms pitta and stimulates kapha. Brings stability, groundedness and wisdom.	Jupiter
Red Coral (pravāla)	Sweet and pungent, cooling, sweet. Strength giving. Regulates pitta, neutral for vāta and kapha. Improves color complexion and imparts gracefulness to the person.	Mars
Diamond (vajra)	Pungent and astringent, heating, pungent. Tridoshic, but may disturb some pitta people. Brings prosperity. Strengthens shukra. Improves romantic qualities, digestion, and slows aging.	Venus
Blue Sapphire (nīlam)	Pungent, heating, pungent. Calms vāta and kapha, stimulates pitta. Gives energy to the nerves, bones, joints and muscles.	Saturn
Lapis Lazuli (indranīla)	Bitter, cooling, sweet. Calms vāta and pitta, stimulates kapha. Good for liver and gallbladder, regulates bile. Also good for skin disease.	Saturn-like energy

Table 9: Gemstones and Their Effects

GEMSTONE	EFFECT	PLANET
Emerald (harinmani)	Sweet, cooling, sweet. Calms vāta and pitta, may stimulate kapha. Removes nervousness, improves writing and lecturing skills, gives intelligence.	Mercury
Moonstone (vaidūrya, lasnya)	Pungent, heating, pungent. Calms vāta and kapha, stimulates pitta. Produces energy, cures cold, renal disorder. Good for diabetes and arthritis.	Ketu
Sūryākānta	Sweet, heating, sweet. Pacifies vāta and kapha, may stimulate pitta. Stops bleeding, improves memory and helps seizures.	Sun-like energy
Quartz Crystals (sphatika)	Pungent and sweet, cooling, sweet. Calms vāta, stimulates pitta and kapha. Good for gas, fistula. Improves communication and enhances intuition.	Venus-like energy
Onyx (tribhuja, harita pīta mani)	Pungent, heating, pungent. Calms vāta and kapha, may aggravate pitta. Good for epilepsy, Parkinson's disease, schizophrenia. Improves love and positive thinking.	Sun- and Jupiter-like energy
Bloodstone (lohita, jyotirāja)	Sour and pungent, heating, pungent. Calms vāta and kapha, stimulates pitta. Good for anemia, improves agni, heals stomach ulcer, improves memory. Gives energy, warmth, improves circulation and builds liver and gallbladder energy.	Mars- and Sun-like energy
Jade (nephrite, yashava, bhisma pashan)	Sour and pungent, slightly heating, pungent. Calms vāta and kapha, stimulates pitta. Good for prostate and kidney disease.	Mercury-like energy
Amethyst (nīla sphatika)	Sweet, cooling, sweet. Tridoshic. For mental clarity. Acts on majjā dhātu. Helps neuromuscular weakness.	Saturn-like energy
Opal (sāgararāja, varuna)	Sweet, cooling, sweet. Stimulates vāta and kapha, calms pitta. Improves vision and relieves fever. Enhances spiritual feelings and unfolds intuition. Good for migraine headache.	Neptune-like energy
Alexandrite (hemaratna, harshal)	Sweet and sour, cooling, sweet. Stimulates vāta and kapha, pacifies pitta. Brings tranquility and enhances memory.	Uranus-like energy
Aquamarine (harita nīla mani)	Sweet and astringent, cooling, sweet. Tridoshic. Eliminates dullness of mind and brings mental happiness and intelligence. Enhances love in relationship.	Venus-like energy

9

OTHER PULSE TYPES AND PULSE IN PROGNOSIS

In addition to the commonly used radial pulse, it is also possible to feel the pulse in the temporal region on the side of the head. In some people the temporal pulse moves in a zigzag fashion. When the right brain is functionally active, there is more female energy and a clear throb can be felt on the right side. When the left brain is working, which is male energy, a prominent throb on the left side is experienced. If one keeps a record of the temporal pulse in the morning, afternoon and evening, and continually gets throbbing on the middle finger on the right temporal artery, that person is prone to migraine. In every migraine headache, pitta dosha is a cause, while vāta or kapha may be involved as the secondary dosha.

If throbbing under the index finger at the site of the temporal pulse is felt more on the left side of the head, the person has poor memory caused by vāta. But feel it morning, afternoon and evening for eight days in a row. A consistent reading indicates that this person is losing either recent or remote memory. Vāta will be high and is responsible for majjā dhātu's loss of memory, which may even lead to dementia. If kapha is the predominant pulse, either on the right or the left side of the head, tarpaka kapha is aggravated and may lead to manic depression. So for the temporal pulse, a vāta pulse shows pre-dementia, a pitta pulse shows migraine, and a kapha pulse shows bipolar or manic depression.

There are other pulses—the orbital pulse, carotid pulse and brachial pulse. If the radial pulse is feeble and there is a strong brachial pulse, the patient will be all right for five years. The brachial pulse is the pulse for longevity. If the radial pulse is feeble and the left brachial artery is thin, slender and elastic, that means the person will have a favorable prognosis for more than five years.

Feel the axillary pulse under the armpits. This pulse is called *jīvana darshani*, the "don't worry, be happy" pulse. If this pulse is strong and feels like a long slender cord, that person has a tendency for long life. However, disease pathology is invasive and the person may become fatally ill at any moment, even though the pulses are strong. If there is no pulse in between the eyebrows (orbital pulse), the person may become sick within six weeks. The pulse at the eyebrows is connected to the immune system.

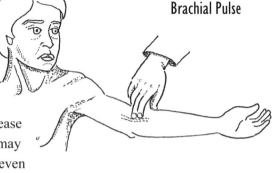

Brachial Pulse

Axillary Pulse

There are a few other interesting pulses. In a pitta person, lack of a strong throbbing of the pitta pulse in the posterior tibial artery on the right foot means the person may become sick within one month. If the posterior tibial artery is extremely feeble on the left foot, then a kapha person may become sick. One month is not a fixed period, but is only approximate. If the posterior tibial pulse is not perceptible at all during a serious illness, it denotes that the patient will live only for a day or two.

The orbital pulse is felt between the thumb and index fingers.

In a vāta person, if the dorsalis pedis artery on the top of the arch is extremely weak, that person will be sick within one month. Compare on both feet. This pulse is important in assessing the circulation of the lower extremities in post-operative cases as well as in cases of gangrene.

Posterior Tibial Artery

Dorsalis Pedis Artery

If the posterior tibial artery pulse is very feeble and imperceptible, it indicates serious illness with a bad prognosis.

Gangrenous Tissue

Blockage of the Blood Vessel

The concept of nādi in the ancient Vedas is much more than the physical arteries. The rishis' concept of nādi includes the flow of prāna that is moving through the body. The physio-pathological changes of these pranic currents, etheric channels of energy moving through the cardiovascular system, can best be felt through the radial, brachial, axillary, carotid, temporal, femoral, dorsalis pedis and posterior tibial arteries, and these are the locations where we can feel the pulse.

✧   The radial pulse is the one most commonly felt.
✧   The temporal pulse can be read during complaints of dizziness, fits, Parkinson's, migraine headache, sinus conditions, poor memory and insomnia. The functions of prāna vāyu, sādhaka pitta and tarpaka kapha can be checked at this location.
✧   The carotid pulse should be felt in hyper- and hypothyroidism, laryngitis, pharyngitis, speech disorders and during shock and unconsciousness. The carotid pulse is located close to the heart and indicates the activities of udāna vāyu and prāna vāyu.
✧   The brachial pulse is felt during pleurisy, pericarditis, diabetes and generalized anasarca. This pulse indicates the activities of avalambaka kapha and kledaka kapha.
✧   The abdominal pulse is felt when there is abdominal discomfort, diarrhea, dysentery or sprue syndrome. Samāna vāyu and pāchaka pitta can be checked at this site.
✧   The thumb pulse is felt in cases of massive edema, when the radial or brachial pulses cannot be felt. It is connected to vyāna vāyu, prāna vāyu and kledaka kapha.
✧   The femoral pulse is felt during pelvic, bladder, uterine, testicular and ovarian disorders. This pulse is related to apāna vāyu activity. In aortic regurgitation the femoral pulse becomes heaving and creates a sound like a pistol shot which can be heard through the stethoscope.
✧   The popliteal pulse is felt in solid edema, lymphatic edema and arthritis. It is connected to vyāna vāyu and lymphatic circulation.
✧   The posterior tibial pulse is felt when there is edema on the legs, nephrotic syndrome or kidney disorder. This pulse indicates the activity of kledaka kapha and apāna vāyu.
✧   The dorsalis pedis pulse is felt to confirm the circulation of the lower extremities in post-operative and pre-gangrenous conditions. This pulse indicates the activity of vyāna vāyu, kledaka kapha and prāna vāyu.
✧   All of these pulses can be used to confirm conditions detected in the radial pulse and to check the activities of the doshic sub types.

THE PULSE IN PROGNOSIS

The ancient sūtras contain knowledge about using the pulse to gain information about what will happen to the patient. Some of these sūtras even reveal information about the pulse showing how long the person will live and how much chance of recovery he or she has. At this point we will switch our attention to using the pulse in prognosis.

First, we will consider pulse conditions with favorable prognosis. If the radial pulse at all levels beats for 30 beats in its own place, with regularity in rhythm and consistent strength and volume, the patient is assured of longevity. This pulse is called *dīrghāyushya* (long life pulse).

If the pulse is not displaced from its own site and seems to be flexible, there is no fear of death and the disease will be cured.

If the prakruti (deep) and vikruti (superficial) pulses both show the same qualities and dosha spikes, the prognosis is good.

If the pulse beats like the progression of a quail at the site of pitta and at the time of pitta, it indicates good health. If the pulse beats like the progression of a swan or partridge at the site of kapha and at the time of kapha, it indicates good health. Similarly, if the pulse beats like the progression of a cobra during vāta time, the condition is also favorable.

We can examine all seven levels of the pulse in a normal healthy person, but when a person is extremely sick in the bheda stage, the seventh level of the pulse is extremely feeble. This means that the vikruti pulse is encroaching on the prakruti. In that condition, the prognosis is not good. The life governing factors are ojas, tejas and prāna, which can be felt in the fourth level pulse. When ojas and tejas are totally depleted and only prāna is present, one can feel the fourth level pulse only under the index finger. That means that the person is living on only prāna and it is a fatal condition.

Wide gap between two uplifts.

When a patient is dying, the pulse is not present in all seven levels and there is only an ant-like movement under the seventh level. In that condition, don't go into superficial and deep levels, but just try to feel the pulse in general, as its nature is very subtle. Just a little pulsation comes along, then a bit more comes. The pulse is like a thread and each throb has distance from the next. There is a wide gap between two uplifts and it comes up and disappears. The throbs have clarity and a steep stroke, quick and soft, and can only be felt under the index finger. Such a pulse indicates an unfavorable condition and the patient's life is in danger.

The next pulse to consider is extremely faint. It comes for a few beats and then there is a gap, a couple of faint uplifts and then another gap. It is irregu-

Faint uplifts with gaps between them.

larly irregular; a soft, slow, agitated pulse. This pulse shows a tridoshic involvement and is also a quite serious and unfavorable condition.

In some patients, the radial pulse is completely absent and only the carotid can be felt. The carotid is called *jīvana sakshi*, life witnessing, and it shows the presence of life. If three fingers are placed on the carotid, with the vāta finger at the distal position, and the pulse is only delicately felt under the ring finger, this means the person's life will last for only 12 hours.

What are the conditions when the pulse becomes imperceptible? The pulse is difficult to find in trauma or shock, either psychological or physical. The cardinal signs of shock are perspiration, pulselessness (which means imperceptible pulse), pallor and falling blood pressure. Other precipitating conditions include suffering from a fall, fright and fainting.

Carotid Pulse

Vāta spike under the index finger indicates impaired function.
Pitta spike under the middle finger denotes overactive function.
Kapha spike under the ring finger shows underactive function.

Other examples include cholera, where the pulse becomes impalpable because of severe dehydration. Also, when a bone is fractured, causing blood to go to the area of the injury, the pulse is difficult to feel. Other conditions of impalpable pulse are severe diarrhea and vomiting, which also lead to dehydration. In influenza, when a person perspires too much, the pulse is faint. In addition, hypothermia, multiple orgasms in one night and severe blood loss will all affect the pulse. Sushruta was a surgeon and comments about the effect of blood loss can be found in his writings.

Coma

The pulse of a person in a coma will vary depending upon the type of coma. If it is a diabetic coma, the pulse may be of two types. The first is hyperglycemia, in which the pulse will be like kapha—slow, steady, deep, heavy—and will be felt only under the ring finger. The second is hypoglycemia, in which case the index finger pulse will show vāta characteristics.

In hepatic pre-coma, the patient is rowdy and violent, and says nonsensical things, because the toxins from the liver are affecting the higher cerebral centers. When a person goes into a hepatic coma, it is difficult to bring that person back to consciousness. The pulse has a pitta nature, bounding and jumping like an angry frog. However the patient is totally unconscious and doesn't respond even to painful stimuli. Uremic coma is brought on by renal failure with high urea levels in the blood. Toxins from the kidneys lodge in the lungs and brain, causing the person to have severe breathlessness. The pulse will have vāta and pitta characteristics. A coma due to encephalitis, which is a viral infection, will create pitta and kapha spikes in the pulse. Tarpaka kapha and sādhaka pitta are affected. Finally, a meningeal coma will manifest an extremely feeble vāta type pulse.

Unfavorable Prognosis

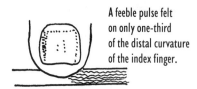

A feeble pulse felt on only one-third of the distal curvature of the index finger.

When a patient is confined to bed and the pulse under the index finger is felt on only one-third of the distal curvature, that is a most serious condition.

If the pulse under each finger (index, middle and ring) is displaced from its normal position, it indicates an unfavorable prognosis. This pulse shows displaced ojas (*ojo visramsa*). However in some individuals, one has to consider the possibility of a congenitally displaced pulse, called normal anatomical disposition. This is not pathological.

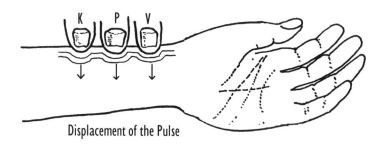

Displacement of the Pulse

The pulse that stops and beats slowly and then stops again indicates a fatal condition (complete heart block). This pulse indicates depleted prāna.

The pulse that is very cold to the touch and nearly imperceptible indicates poor vyāna and is generally a fatal condition. This pulse indicates myocardial failure and vasomotor paresis.

The pulse that is deep-seated and extremely feeble indicates that death is approaching.

The pulse that is irregular, feeble, deep and felt only between two fingers indicates a very serious condition and is considered hopeless.

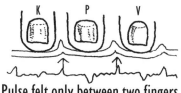

Pulse felt only between two fingers.

If the pulse leaves its normal site, disappears and then immediately comes back again to that same site, such a pulse indicates death is near.

The pulse that jumps like a sparrow indicates the condition will be curable only with prolonged and difficult effort.

If the pulse is cool, weak and like a soft thread, it indicates death. This is an ill-defined pulse due to weak heart and relaxed vascular tension.

If the pulse beats with extreme rapidity, it indicates a bad prognosis.

If the pulse beats like the progression of a frog at one time, like that of a swan at another time and then becomes rapid like a snake for a moment, and if the patient has had a fever for one month or so, that indicates triple doshic derangement and there is no hope of life. An example of this condition is toxemia due to typhoid fever or perforated peritonitis. This pulse is true of typhoid fever, even though in the beginning of this condition there is relative bradycardia (slow pulse).

If the pitta pulse under the middle finger becomes snake-like, the kapha pulse under the ring finger becomes coil-like, and the vāta pulse under the index finger becomes zigzagged and crooked, that means death will occur in four days.

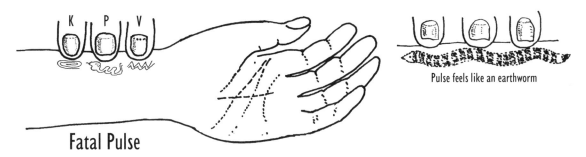

Fatal Pulse

Pulse feels like an earthworm

If the pulse beats like the progression of an earthworm and again like a snake, and feels slender and fine, that indicates that the patient will die at the end of a month's time.

Pulse Conditions with Unfavorable Prognosis

The following pulse conditions are indicative of bad prognosis:

- ✧ Increased rapidity of the pulse
- ✧ Hardness (this indicates that the pulse is felt between the beats, as in arteriosclerosis)
- ✧ Extreme slowness of the pulse (due to heart block)
- ✧ High tension pulse (hypertension)
- ✧ Extreme smallness (dehydration)
- ✧ Extreme arrhythmia (multiple extra systole)
- ✧ Displacement of the pulse from its normal site
- ✧ Imperceptible pulse
- ✧ Irregularly irregular pulse (atrial flutter with fibrillation)
- ✧ A pulse that is only felt under the index finger at the vāta spike, is very feeble and moves like an ant.

Summary

Āyurveda says logic gives discriminating capacity and physical proof. Therefore, logic is welcome. But there are many things that cannot be proven on the physical level. Physical proof based upon objectivity is limited. Subjective experience is vast, and that is why every individual is an authority when telling exactly how he or she experiences something. In pulse diagnosis, the patient is also an authority, because it is the patient who first realizes the symptoms and then tells the physician. Then the physician observes, examines and comes to an understanding of the etiology and pathogenesis of the condition. To describe experience accurately demands a great deal of awareness. Nādi vijñānam, the ancient art of pulse in Āyurveda, is based upon both subjective experience and objective observation.

There is an ancient book called *Yoga Vāsishtha*. In that text, Rāma's guru, Vashishtha, gives a dialogue about nādi vijñānam. There, he names the major nādis including those mentioned earlier in this text. An additional nādi is sushumnā, the spinal cord, which has no pulsation and is not directly related to the cardiovascular pulse. It is a main nerve, even though it is called a nādi. *Īdā* is the left sympathetic trunk and *pingalā* is the right trunk connected to the spinal cord. *Brahma randhra*, located at the anterior fontanel of the brain, is connected to īdā. Shiva randhra, located at the posterior fontanel, is related to pingalā.

Within the sushumnā there is an important nādi called chitrā. When this nādi is activated, the central canal of the spinal cord gives higher spiritual vision, which is the meaning of chitrā. It is full of beauty and awareness and leads to *brahma nādi*, which is located at the foramen lacerum, a small aperture in the brain. Other nādis are *vilambikā*, the sciatic nerve, and sarasvatī, the lingual nerve. The goddess of language is Sarasvatī, and under the tongue there is a network of nerves called *lalanā chakra*, which is related to *sarasvatī nādi*. *Pūsha nādi* is related to the left ear and *gandharī nādi* to the right ear. The *alambushā nādi* is connected to the reproductive organs, penis and vagina.

We cannot feel these nādis, because they are subtle and deep. These nādis are not palpated by Āyurvedic physicians for diagnostic purposes. They are awakened through meditation and yogic practice. Our objective is to awaken sushumnā, chitrā and brahma nādis and become enlightened, but mere intellectual knowledge of the yogic nādis is not going to make life complete. Knowing oneself through the practical application of the radial pulse is essential. To know one's self is to know one's prakruti and vikruti, and this self-knowing is the foundation of life. For that purpose, one has to master the radial pulse.

One can develop extrasensory perception through meditation and daily practice of reading the pulse, and with the grace of God. It is practice which brings perfection. You are the best book, you are your teacher, your disciple, your student, your friend and your guru. Learn from your observations. Read all seven levels of your own pulse and keep a record. One day you will receive the gift of grace and the doors of perception will open.

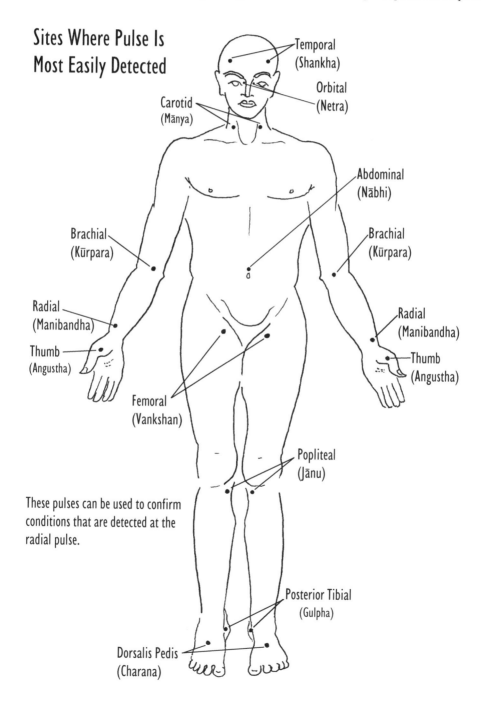

Sites Where Pulse Is Most Easily Detected

Temporal (Shankha)

Orbital (Netra)

Carotid (Mānya)

Abdominal (Nābhi)

Brachial (Kūrpara)

Brachial (Kūrpara)

Radial (Manibandha)

Radial (Manibandha)

Thumb (Angustha)

Thumb (Angustha)

Femoral (Vankshan)

Popliteal (Jānu)

These pulses can be used to confirm conditions that are detected at the radial pulse.

Posterior Tibial (Gulpha)

Dorsalis Pedis (Charana)

The Seven Levels of the Pulse

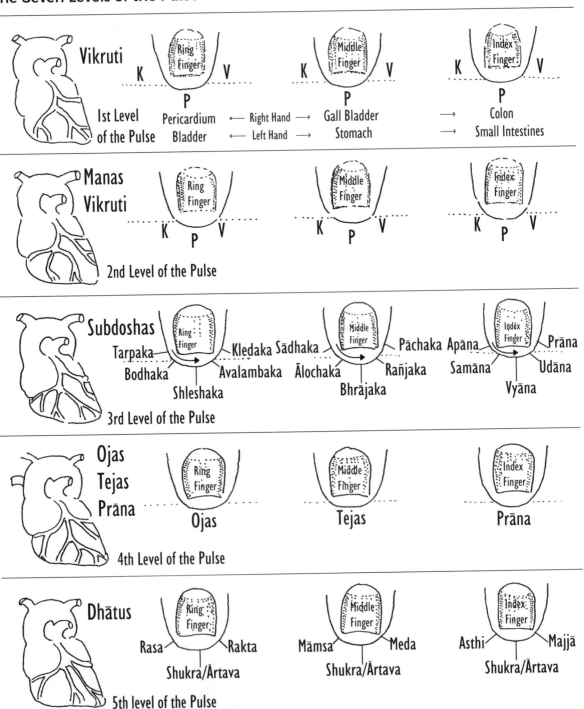

Vikruti

K — Ring Finger — V
P
1st Level of the Pulse   Pericardium   ← Right Hand →   Gall Bladder
Bladder   ← Left Hand →   Stomach

K — Middle Finger — V
P

K — Index Finger — V
P
→   Colon
→   Small Intestines

Manas Vikruti

Ring Finger
K   P   V
2nd Level of the Pulse

Middle Finger
K   P   V

Index Finger
K   P   V

Subdoshas

Tarpaka — Ring Finger — Kledaka Sādhaka
Bodhaka   Avalambaka
Shleshaka
3rd Level of the Pulse

Pāchaka Apāna — Middle Finger — Rañjaka
Ālochaka   Samāna
Bhrājaka

Prāna — Index Finger
Udāna
Vyāna

Ojas Tejas Prāna

Ring Finger
Ojas
4th Level of the Pulse

Middle Finger
Tejas

Index Finger
Prāna

Dhātus

Rasa — Ring Finger — Rakta
Shukra/Ārtava
5th level of the Pulse

Māmsa — Middle Finger — Meda
Shukra/Ārtava

Asthi — Index Finger — Majjā
Shukra/Ārtava

The Seven Levels of the Pulse

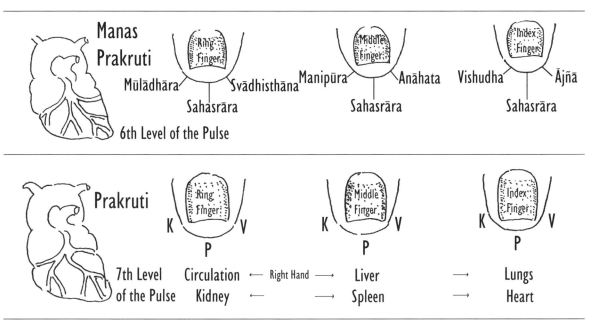

GLOSSARY

A

āhāra rasa — the end product of digested food that nourishes all bodily tissues; chyle

ājñā — the center point between the eyebrows where right meets with left, alpha meets with omega, and intuition meets with logic; it is the highest end point of human polarity

ākruti — the volume and tension of the pulse

ālochaka pitta — one of the subtypes of pitta, situated in the sense organ of seeing; it is responsible for vision and color perception

āma — the raw, undigested food products that, having become fetid, become toxic to the system; the root cause of many diseases

āma vāta — rheumatoid arthritis (vāta carrying āma into the joints)

āmāshaya — the stomach as a vessel of undigested food

ārtava dhātu — one of the seven dhātus (bodily tissues); the female reproductive tissue; ova, the female eggs

āshaya — a vessel

Āyurveda — the science of life; its roots are in the Sanskrit words "ayur" meaning life and "veda" meaning the ancient scriptures roughly translated as knowledge or science

adha jatru granthi — the thymus gland

agni — the fire element in the body that regulates body heat and performs digestion, absorption and assimilation of food stuff. It transforms food into energy or consciousness.

Agni — a type of individual personality that, when detected at the sixth level of the pulse, indicates a worshipper of knowledge

ahamkāra — a continuous feeling of "I am"; a center in the daily operating consciousness from where each individual thinks, feels and acts

alambushā nādi — connected to the reproductive organs

ambu vaha srotas — water-regulating channels of the body connected to the gastrointestinal mucous membrane and indirectly connected to the organs of water, the kidney and sweat glands, and includes the cerebro-spinal fluid as well.

anāhata — the heart chakra; the center of unconditional love in the heart, it also denotes the cardiac plexus which governs heart activity.

angustha purusha — a mystic, thumb-sized flame of individual consciousness that can be seen at the right chamber of the heart during deep meditation

añjali — a measurement formed when two hands meet together to make an empty bowl.

antar darshana — inner vision or insight

anuchāra — beyond the power of speech where words cannot reach, where thoughts cannot describe; this point is located about the width of 10 fingers above the physical brain; it is the junction between the auric field and cosmic consciousness

apāna — to eliminate

apāna vāyu — one of the subtypes of vāta that regulates excretion, elimination and downward movement

asthi bhagna — a bone fracture

asthi dhātu — one of the seven dhātus; the bone tissue which supports the body, giving protection, shape and longevity

asthi saushiryam — osteoporosis

aum — the primordial cosmic soundless sound; it is written as a-u-m which represents creation, preservation and transformation of everything that exists in form or that can be expressed by experience

avabāhuka — acute arthritis of the shoulder joint; a pain in the neck, shoulder and along the arm due to a pinched nerve(s)

avalambaka kapha — one of the five kapha subtypes present in the heart and lungs that supports all bodily kapha through circulation

B

bala — the force or strength of the pulse

basti — one of the five important cleansing measures of pañchakarma; it eliminates excess vāta dosha out of the system via medicated herbal tea or oil enemas and normalizes all *vāta* disorders

bhagandara — fistula in ano

bhairavī mudrā — also called shāmbhavī mudrā, a practice of looking at an outer object while at the same time looking at the inner looker; this practice gradually develops into passive awareness and a witnessing state of bliss

bhakti — the love divine that is felt in the heart center

bhakti yoga — one of the spiritual paths of yoga, the path of devotion leading to oneness with the Divine within one's self

bhasma — a specialized Āyurvedic compound alchemically prepared by proper purification and burning into ash; bhasmas have a high potency and release prāna into the system

bhastrikā — a breathing practice where air is passively drawn in and forcibly pushed out, as in a bellows; a practice to increase heat and improve circulation

bheda — the seventh stage of the disease process, complete manifestation, where one can differentiate the disease; during this stage the involvement of each dhātu is clearly differentiated with its complications and structural changes

bhisma pashan — jade

bhrājaka pitta — one of the five subtypes of pitta, located in the skin of the entire body; its function is to give tactile sensation, color complexion and luster to the skin

bhrāmarī — a type of breathing exercise where a soft humming sound, like a bee, is made during exhalation and/or during inhalation; a practice for calming the mind and sādhaka pitta in the system

bhūta agni — present in the liver and gastrointestinal tract and governing the transformation of the elements of Ether, Air, Fire, Water, and Earth present in food into the biological elements. For each element there is a specific bhūta agni.

bhūtonmāda — psychosis due to the influence of an evil spirit

bīja mantra — a sacred, subtle, primordial sound from a Sanskrit word associated with the chakras

bodhaka kapha — one of the five subtypes of kapha; located in the mouth, tongue and larynx, it enables the perception of taste and assists in digestion

Brahma — the pure, expansive, all-pervasive universal consciousness; sattvic, creative potential; one of the three aspects of the Hindu trinity of God

brahma nādi — located at the foramen lacerum, a small aperture in the brain

brahma randhra — a small opening in the cranium, located at the anterior fontanel of the brain and connected to cosmic consciousness

C

chakras — the energy centers in the body; related to nerve plexus centers which govern the bodily functions. Each chakra is a separate reservoir of consciousness connecting the physical body to the astral body.

chidākāsha — a space within the brain that is functionally connected to the synaptic spaces in between the neurons; the inner space of pure awareness present in the ventricles of the brain

chitrā nādi — a nādi at the central canal of the spinal cord that, when activated, gives higher spiritual vision full of beauty and awareness; a bridge between the physical and astral bodies, expressed in the fifth level of the pulse

D

darshana — observation; looking for the signs and symptoms of disease by the process of observation; a total seeing without comparison and judgment; being in the presence of someone

dhārana — the mental contemplation and retention of information into memory

dhāranī — that which holds all organs together

dhātu — "dha" means to hold together, to build together; dhātu is the structural, building, elemental tissue; there are seven tissues defined in Āyurveda: rasa (plasma), rakta (blood tissue), māmsa (muscle tissue), meda (adipose tissue), asthi (bone marrow), majjā (bone and nerves), shukra (male reproductive tissue) and ārtava (female reproductive tissue).

dhātu agni — the fire element within each dhātu responsible for the selection of proper nutrient substances, according to the specific dhātu's needs, and the transformation of nutrient substances appropriate to the corresponding dhātu and each dhātu's by-products, waste products and the next dhātu's immature tissue; keeps the dhātu healthy and functioning properly

dhātu kalā — a membranous structure that surrounds each tissue, separating it from the adjacent tissue. Within each kalā, that dhātu's agni, ojas, tejas and prāna are located and perform the normal functions of the tissue independent of the other dhātu kalās.

dhamanī — a pulsating blood vessel or artery

dhanustambha — tetanus

dīrghāyushya — a type of pulse indicating long life

dosha — referring to vāta, pitta and kapha; the main three psycho-physiological functional principles of the body which determine each individual's constitution at the time of conception. The doshas govern the individual's response to changes when they are normal. When disturbed, they can initiate the disease process.

doshic — referring to one or more of the three doshas

drava — liquid

G

gaja gati — the elephant pulse; shows extremely high kapha blocked in the lymphatic tissue; this pulse is present under the kapha finger

gandakāla — an indication or warning of a critical illness, calamity or accident of the future that is felt only in the fifth level pulse

gandharī nādi — related to the right ear

garbha gulma — a state where the cells of the uterus lose their intelligence and think that the uterus has conceived, continuing to grow; as in a uterine fibroid tumor

garbhā sravanam — miscarriage

gati — the manner in which the pulse moves; the pulse is described by comparing it to the movements of different animals

gatī yantra grahani — chronic malabsorption syndrome; tuberculosis of the small intestine

ghee — clarified butter

graha chikitsā — astrotherapy using the healing influences of the planets and their gemstones, crystals and mantras

grahani — chronic diarrhea, malabsorption syndrome in the small intestine

granthi roga — lymphadenitis

granthi rupā nādi — syphilitic arteriosclerosis

gulma — any tumor, lump or diverticulosis

guna — three qualities influencing all creation: sattva, rajas and tamas. Sattvic qualities imply essence, reality, consciousness, purity and clarity of perception. All movement and activities are due to rajas. Tamasic qualities bring darkness, inertia, heaviness and materialistic attitudes. There is a constant interplay of these three gunas in all creation.

guru — teacher; one who removes the darkness of ignorance; the channel through which knowledge of God comes to one; also, heavy, an attribute characterized by heaviness, weight and bulk

H

halimaka — malignant jaundice or hepatitis C

ham — the mantra of the fifth chakra, the throat chakra, vishuddha; the seed sound of the space element

hamsa — a male swan; the sound vibrations of the breath that make up the sound of the "so-hum" mantra, "so" during inhalation and "hum" during exhalation. "So" represents cosmic consciousness and "hum" the individual ego.

hamsa gati — the swan pulse, the primary description of the kapha pulse

hamsī — a female swan; also the sound vibrations of the breath moving through the pulse; a synonym for the pulse

Hanuman Chalisa — the 40 poetic, sacred mantras for praying to the eternal, ever-living servant of Ram, Hanuman, the model of devotion and service

hanustambha — lockjaw

harinmani — an emerald gemstone

harita nīla mani — an aquamarine gemstone

harita pīta mani — onyx

harshal — an Alexandrite gemstone

hemaratna — an Alexandrite gemstone

hrid roga — heart disease

hridaya dhārā kala — the membranous structure around the heart; i.e., the pericardium and endocardium

I

īdā — the subtle energy channel which flows along the left side of sushumnā and controls the parasympathetic branch of the autonomic nervous system

Indra — a personality type, found at the sixth level of the pulse, indicating a royal and religious personality

indranīla — lapis lazuli

Ishānya — a personality type, found at the sixth level of the pulse, indicating someone who is sattvic, fortunate and spiritual

J

jāthara agni — the digestive fire, located in the duodenum and the stomach; the central fire of the body; responsible for the digestion and transformation of food materials

jīva — the individual consciousness, soul; a reflection of the divine

jīvana darshani — axillary pulse under the armpits; the "don't worry, be happy" pulse

jñāna yoga — one of the three main spiritual paths, the path of knowledge to realize God or the Divine within one's self

jyotirāja — bloodstone

jyotish — Vedic astrology

K

kāka — a crow, used to describe a type of pitta pulse

kāla — time; a movement of prāna; respiration rate of 12-15 breaths per minute

kāmala — jaundice or hepatitis A

kāsa — cough

kāthinya — the consistency or hardening of the blood vessel wall

kalā — the membranous structure that holds a tissue, separating one from the other; it also lines all organs and cavities in the body

kampa vāta — Parkinson's disease or vepathu

kanda — a prolapsed uterus

kapha — one of the three doshas, combining the water and earth elements; the energy which forms the body's structure—bones, muscles, tendons—and provides the "glue" that holds the cells together. Kapha supplies the water for all bodily parts and systems. It lubricates joints, moisturizes the skin, and maintains immunity. In balance, kapha is expressed as love, calmness and forgiveness. Out of balance, it leads to attachment, greed and envy.

kapha gulma — any encapsulated benign tumor, cystic swelling or ameboma creating a tumor-like structure

karma yoga — one of the three main spiritual paths, a path of action for attaining liberation

khavaigunya — a weak or defective space within an organ or tissue of the body where a pathological condition is likely to begin

kledaka kapha — one of the kapha subtypes; its function is to moisten the food particles; after breaking them into small pieces, it liquefies the digested contents of food materials in the stomach and protects the stomach wall from the digestive enzymes and acids; active in the stomach

kloma — pancreas and caudate plexus in the brain which secretes cerebrospinal fluid and is the root of ambu vaha srotas

kosha — sheath; subtle body; there are five sheaths: sheath of bliss, sheath of knowledge, sheath of mind, sheath of prāna and sheath of food.

kshaya — diminished, deteriorated, deficient or decreased

Kubera — a personality type, found at the sixth level of the pulse, indicating someone who is sattvic, rich in mind and blessed with long life

kundalinī — a coiled, serpentine spiritual energy which, for most people, is dormant at the root of the spine

kundalinī shakti — the power of pure energy; the term used in speaking of the awakening of spiritual energies

L

lāvaka — the common quail, used to describe a type of pitta pulse

laghu — light; an attribute characterized by aiding digestion and cleansing, promoting freshness and alertness. In excess, it may cause insomnia and ungroundedness.

lalanā chakra — the sublingual lower plexus or network of nerves under the tongue that controls the movements of the tongue and helps in speech

lam — the mantra of the first chakra, mūlādhāra, the seed sound of the earth element

lasnya — moonstone gemstone

lohita — bloodstone; also means iron-containing liquid connective tissue; the blood

Lord Shiva — the third God in the Hindu Godhead Trinity; the deity of the people, of the common folk; literally, Shiva means "good" or "auspicious"; known as Rudra, the dissolver, the benevolent one; Shiva has eight qualities: independence, purity, self-knowledge, omniscience, freedom from mala, boundless benevolence, omnipotence, and bliss

M

mālā — a string of beads for mantra, prayer and other devotional practices

māmsa dhārā kalā — a membranous structure which is the muscle sheath that separates one muscle from another

māmsa dhātu — one of the seven dhātus; the muscle tissue; produced by rasa and rakta, its main function is to provide physical strength, coordination, movement, covering, form and protection.

madhumeha — glycosuria; juvenile diabetes or diabetes insipidus

Mahad — the great principle; intelligence, the cosmic aspect of the intellect, containing also the individual intellect, called Buddhi, ego and mind, it is present in the creation of the universe. Its special function is determination.

Mahesvara — tamas, resistance to change or potential destructive force

majjā dhātu — one of the seven dhātus; the bone marrow and nerve tissue; it is unctuous and soft; its main function is to oleate the body, to fill up the bone, and to nourish shukra dhātu. It plays an important role in communication.

malas — any impurity, the waste products produced in the body through the processes of digestion; malas must constantly be moving out of the body as they are produced.

manda — slow; characterized by slow action, sluggishness, dullness, relaxation

manda agni — a condition of agni, slow gastric fire; kapha-type fire, resulting in slow digestion and slow metabolism

mandūka gati — the frog pulse; the primary description of the pitta pulse

manika — a ruby gemstone

manipūra — the third chakra, located in the region of the solar plexus and umbilicus

mantra — a sacred word or phrase of spiritual significance and power; mantras are of two classes: 1) those given expression by the voice and 2) those that are not spoken but listened to internally. Every mantra has its own deity, meter and rishi, the observer.

mantra yoga — union with God through the power of mantra

mayūra gati — the peacock pulse, common in arterial hypertension; occurs most often in pitta-kapha people

meda dhārā kalā — membranous structure or fascia which holds adipose tissue on the buttocks, belly, chest and the cheeks

meda dhātu — one of the seven bodily tissues; the fat tissue, supported by māmsa dhātu (muscle tissue); the function of meda (fat) is to give shape and to lubricate the body; adipose tissue/fat in excessive quantity may produce obesity and physical weakness

manas — the mind

manas prakruti — the constitution of the mind

manas vikruti — the current state of the mind or the altered state of the mind

moti — a pearl gemstone

mudrā — a gesture or arrangement of the fingers for communication between body, mind and consciousness

mukha pāka — stomatitis or ulcer

mūlādhāra — the first chakra, located in the root area of the trunk of the body; associated with survival, groundedness, stability, security and instincts

mūtrakrichra — strangury; dysuria or difficulty in passing urine

mūtrāshaya — the urinary bladder

N

nādi — literally, a river; the river of life as expressed through the pulse; the pulse; a subtle channel

nādi shodana — alternate nostril breathing

nādi vijñānam — the art or science of reading the pulse to detect existing and potential states of a person's body, mind and spirit

Nairutya — a personality type, found at the sixth level of the pulse, indicating someone who is tamasic and loves to sleep

nephrite — jade

nīla sphatika — an amethyst gemstone

nīla shveta mandala — a blue sclera which is present in cases of osteoporosis

nīlam — a blue sapphire gemstone

O

ojas — the pure essence of all bodily tissues (dhātus); the superfine essence of kapha; maintains immunity, strength and vitality of the body. Severe depletion of ojas can lead to the death of the person.

ojo visramsa — displaced ojas; ojas remains unstable during the seventh and eighth months of pregnancy, moving between the body of the fetus and the body of the mother. If a baby is born with insufficient ojas or displaced ojas during the seventh or eighth month, this premature baby's survival is difficult because of the displaced ojas.

P

pāchaka pitta — one of the five subtypes of pitta located in an area between the stomach and the small intestine. It is the combination of bile and pancreatic juices. When functioning abnormally, it may increase the appetite, cause a burning sensation, thirst, insomnia, digestive disorders, diarrhea and/or jaundice.

padma gati — the lotus pulse; a unique pulse indicating that the person is enlightened; felt under the kapha finger

padmarāga mani — a ruby gemstone

pakvāshaya shūla — colic

pañchakarma — the five-fold measures for elimination of excess dosha and/or āma from the body. Used for the purpose of internal purification, they are: vomiting (vaman), purgation (virechan), decoction or oil enema (basti), bloodletting (rakta moksha) and nasal administration (nasya) through the administration of specific medications

pīlu pāka — the stage of digestion and assimilation in which the lifeless molecules of food, water and air are transformed into conscious, living cells through the subtle energy of pīlu pāka agni

pingalā — a subtle energy channel that flows along the right side of sushumnā and controls the sympathetic branch of the autonomic nervous system

pippalī — Piper longum; a close relative to black pepper that has many medicinal properties, especially for digestion and respiration; a rejuvenating tonic for the lungs and liver

pithara pāka — the subtle stage of digestion and assimilation where the agni of pithara pāka, located at the nucleus of the cells, transforms and uses the qualities of sattva, rajas and tamas contained within the food for nourishing the mind

pitta — one of the three doshas, corresponding to the elements of fire and water; the body's metabolic system; governs digestion, absorption, assimilation, nutrition, metabolism and body temperature. In balance, pitta promotes understanding and intelligence. Out of balance, pitta arouses anger, hatred and jealousy.

pitta dhārā kalā — the mucous membrane of the stomach and small intestine that secretes hydrochloric acid, digestive enzymes and pāchaka pitta

pitta grahani — chronic dysentery, sprue syndrome

pitta gulma — diverticulitis and polyp

plīhā — the spleen

plīhā roga — splenic disorders

prāna — the vital life energy without which life cannot exist; the flow of cellular intelligence from one cell into another

prāna vaha srotas — the air-carrying channels, consisting of the lungs, heart, all respiratory passages and the colon

prāna vāta, prāna vāyu — a subtype of vāta dosha seated in the brain that governs the higher cerebral activities; moves downward and inward and controls all sensory and mental functions; also responsible for respiratory functions, regulating inhalation

prānāyāma — the control of life-energy by various techniques that regulate and restrain breath through which one can control the mind and improve one's quality of awareness and perception; helps in all types of meditation

prānāchārya — one who heals by balancing the patient's prāna through his or her own *prāna* without using any medicine

prabhāva — the dynamic action of a substance that cannot be explained by the simple logic of its taste, energy and post-digestive effects; the specific action of the herb, medicine or other substance that cannot be explained; electro-magnetic action through the intelligence of the substance

pradara — leukorrhea; a white discharge from the vagina

prakopa — provocation: the second stage in the disease process in which the accumulated dosha rises up from its natural site to affect other organs, e.g., kapha rising up from the stomach to the lungs, causing cough, congestion and excess mucus

prakruti — the psychosomatic, biological constitution of the individual; the fixed constitution of the person established at conception and detected in the deep pulse; inborn tendencies that manifest in the responses of the body and mind to daily living

prasara — the third stage in samprāpti, the disease process, when the aggravated dosha spreads into general circulation, moving into rasa dhātu via the body's normal circulation process

prashna — an art of inquiry and questioning of the patient's personal and family history in order to understand the history of the disease

pratyaksham — what one observes or perceives

pratyaksham alpam — physical proof based upon objectivity

pravāla — red coral

pūjā — a Hindu ritual worship designed to concentrate the mind on God; a ritualistic meditation, done with devotion and affection

Purusha — the higher consciousness that dwells in the "city of the senses" of all beings, which is the physical body

pushkarāja — a yellow sapphire gemstone

R

rāja yakshmā — pulmonary tuberculosis or consumption

Rāma — the seventh incarnation of Vishnu; the warrior-hero of the Rāmāyana; the embodiment of righteousness; also, the mantra of the third chakra, manipūra

rajah — menstruation

rajas — one of the three universal qualities of prakruti, creativity, that which is active, mobile and responsible for movements of sensation

rakta dhārā kalā — the mucous layer or lining of all blood vessels which holds the blood within the arteries and veins

rakta dhātu agni — the heat of the fire element that is present in the blood

rakta dhātu — the second important tissue which mainly contains red blood cells and carries life-energy (prāna) to all bodily tissues, performing the life function, the oxygenation, of all the tissues

rakta vaha srotas — the blood-carrying channels, consisting of the hematopoietic system. Immunologically its function is governed by the liver and spleen.

ram — the mantra of the third chakra, manipūra, located in the region of the solar plexus and umbilicus; the seed sound of the fire element

rañjaka pitta — a pitta subtype; located in the liver and spleen; it confers color and is mainly responsible for the formation of blood, working along with rakta dhātu in the liver and spleen

rasa — the first experience of food stuff in the mouth, e.g., taste. There are six tastes in our diet. Each of these tastes is perceived by different groups of taste buds in the oral cavity.

rasa dhārā kalā — the mucous membrane lining of the lymphatics and veins containing the dhātu agni which transforms food stuff into the bodily lymph and plasma

rasa dhātu — the first of the seven dhātus, rasa is nourished from the digested food and, after absorption, it circulates in the entire body via specific channels; its main function is to provide nutrition to each and every cell of the body; the plasma dhātu

rasāyana — rejuvenation therapy which brings about renewal, regeneration and restoration of all bodily cells, tissues and organs; enhances immunity and stamina, giving longevity to all cells

rishi — a seer; a Vedic sage; the individuals who perceived and/or recorded the Vedic hymns; the enlightened sages who shared their knowledge, medicine, philosophy and religion or spiritual teachings

rishi kesha — a spiritual center located at the top of the fourth ventricle, at the foramen lacerum, where prāna becomes thin like a hair

rutu — the seasons of the year

S

sādhaka pitta — one of the five pitta subtypes; responsible for intelligence, memory and enthusiasm, and is mainly concerned with the functions of the higher mental faculties

sāgararāja — an opal gemstone

Sānkhya — "san" means truth and "khya" means to realize; to realize the theory of the creation of the universe in order to realize the ultimate truth of human life. The term Sānkhya denotes both "discriminative knowledge" and "enumeration"; Sānkhya is one of the schools of Hindu philosophy; founded by Kapila, it gives a systematic account of cosmic evolution according to twenty-five categories: Purusha (Cosmic Spirit), Prakruti (Cosmic Creativity), Mahad (Cosmic Intelligence), Ahamkāra (Individuating Principle), Manas (Mind), Indriyas (Ten Abstract Sense Powers of Cognition and Action), Tanmātrās (Five Subtle Elements), Mahat Bhūtas (The Five Great Elements).

sāra — essence; healthy; the essence of which is characterized by vitality; essential essence of the body; health, as in strong, vigorous, excellent; tissue vitality

sahasrāra — the seventh chakra or crown chakra, located at the topmost part of the skull or head where all polarities end. "Sa" means soma, the lunar energy, "ha" means sun, the male energy. This chakra is where male and female energies merge into one, where the lower meets with the higher, the inner meets with the outer, matter meets with energy, and darkness meets with light, alpha meets with omega, mortality meets with immortality and all definitions dissolve into the undefined.

sama prakruti — the ideal, tridoshic, balanced prakruti; when all the doshas are present equally. Those who have sama prakruti enjoy all seasons and diets, and have long life and perfect health.

samādhi — a state of perfect equilibrium; the balanced state of body, mind and consciousness. "Sama" means balanced, "dhi" means Buddhi. It is a balanced state of supreme intelligence.

samāna — balancing, contracting

samāna vāyu — one of the five vāta subtypes; located in the stomach and small intestine; stimulates agni and digestive enzymes and performs the functions of digestion, absorption and assimilation of food stuff

samprāpti — the pathogenesis of disease; the entire disease process from the cause, etiology, until the complete manifestation of the disease in the bheda stage

sañchaya — the first stage of the disease process, when quantitative accumulation of the dosha takes place

sandhi vāta — osteoarthritis

Sarasvatī — the goddess of speech, the river of learning and the stream of supreme intelligence which is the flow of higher consciousness; the female energy of Brahma

sarasvatī nādi — located at the lingual nerve; see also lalanā chakra

sarita — a river of daily life, a synonym for the pulse

sarpa gati — the cobra pulse; the primary description of the vāta pulse

satyam — timeless, pure existence; it becomes truth

sattva — one of the important gunas of the three qualities of prakruti; denotes light, clarity, purity of perception; the essence of pure awareness.

shāmbhavī mudrā — innocent looking, one is looking without judging, without evaluating, a looking outside at the same time as one is looking inside to the looker; going beyond the object and the looker to the pure state of witnessing awareness which unfolds inner bliss

shāstras — scriptures or scriptural knowledge

shabda tanmātrā — sound; the tanmātrā relating to ether element

shakti — energy; the divine creative will; power, strength

shaktipāta — an energy transmission given by the guru either by touch, by looking into the third eye of the initiate or by reciting mantra, a sacred sound, into the right ear of the disciple so that the inner pure awareness awakens in the heart of the disciple

Shambhu — another name for Lord Shiva, the innocent one

sham-ksham — a merging of the male and female energies at the *ājñā chakra*. The third eye is the meeting point of male and female energies.

shītalī — a practice of prānāyāma (breath control) that cools the system: inhalation is through the curled tongue, with retention; exhalation is slow, steady and complete

Shiva — the Transformer who transforms ego into bliss; the Benevolent One; the Ultimate Reality; good or auspicious; the third in the Hindu God trinity: Brahma, as Creator, Vishnu, as Preserver; Shiva, as Dissolver

shiva randhra — located at the posterior fontanel of the cranium bone and connected to sushumnā nādi

shleshaka kapha — one of the five subtypes of kapha dosha present in all joints which provides lubrication of the joints and gives freedom of movement; also protects the bone from deterioration

shleshma — to hug; the qualities of kapha which hug together and create a compact mass, hence kapha is shleshma

shlīpada — elephantiasis of the leg

shotha — swelling in both feet

shukra dhātu — the seventh tissue; the male reproductive tissue which is white in color, consisting of semen or sperm

shukra or ārtava dhārā kalā — the kalā, producing ojas, that nourishes shukra or ārtava dhātu; present all over the body

shleshma dhārā kalā — the gastric mucous membrane which produces mucosal secretions and protects the stomach wall from burning

snāyu — ligaments that are attached to the muscles and bones at the joints. Their function is to keep the two bones together at the joint.

snigdha — oily; unctuous; soft; characterized by smoothness, moisture, lubrication, vigor, calmness and compassion

so-hum — a mantra used with inhalation and exhalation to enter into meditation; "I am that," beyond limitation of mind and body; the unconscious repetitive prayer that goes on with each inhalation and exhalation of every living creature throughout life. So-hum is the divine sound of universal consciousness occurring in the breath of every being.

soma roga — endometriosis

sparsha — the tactile experience of touch, pain and temperature; one of the eight important examination techniques

sphatika — quartz crystals

srotāmsi (pl.) / srotas (sing.) — the different channels, the special systems. There are innumerable channels in the body; every channel has a root, mula, a passage, marga, and an opening, mukha. Within each channel, the physiological function of the respective organ or system is performed.

stanya — lactation

sthāna samshraya — the fourth stage of samprāpti, the disease process. The site of deposition of dosha and āma where the disease process localizes. This takes place at the site of khavaigunya, defective space; therefore sthāna samshraya becomes the lesion of the disease.

sundaram — beautiful, beauty

sushumnā nādi — the central channel of the spinal cord that carries the kundalinī shakti from the root of the spine to sahasrāra, the crown chakra. The īdā and pingalā nādis are found on each side of sushumnā.

sūryakānta — a special gemstone, pink in color and with the appearance of rose quartz

sūryāvarta — a migraine headache

sūtra — thread, the root of sūtra means to suture; to suture two different ideas, parts or concepts together to create profound meaning

svādhisthāna — the second chakra, located in the pelvic cavity; the seat of self-esteem, courage and self-confidence where vital energy meets with the vital organs

svāti nakshatra — a special star

T

tāla — rhythm; defined as the time interval between two consecutive or successive uplifts of the pulse

tamaka svāsa — bronchial asthma, kapha-type; generally these attacks occur more at night

tamas — one of the three important gunas of prakruti; its characteristics are darkness, inertia and ignorance; responsible for sleep, drowsiness and unconsciousness

tanmātrā — the subtlest part of the five basic elements: sound, touch, sight, taste and smell. Tanmātrās are present in the universe and in the mind of each individual. Through tanmātrā the individual mind experiences the outer object.

tantra — a spiritual path utilizing a set of demanding practices for spiritual growth

tantu — the string of a musical instrument through which one can listen to the music of feelings and emotions, a synonym for the pulse

tapamāna — the temperature of the pulse

tapomani — a gomed gemstone

tarpaka kapha — one of the five kapha subtypes; present in the brain cells as white matter. Within the senses, on the film of tarpaka kapha, all experience, emotions and knowledge are recorded in the form of memory. Therefore tarpaka kapha performs nourishment of all senses, experience and knowledge.

tarpana — the action of a substance, that action being to provide a nutritive, toning, energizing action

tarpanam — nourishing the senses

tejas — the pure essence of the fire element; the superfine essence of pitta dosha which governs the transformation of matter into energy and food, water and air into consciousness

tīkshna — sharp; characterized by penetration, perforation, sharpness, quickness

tīkshna agni — a high metabolism where any quantity of food is digested quickly and the person still remains hungry; a condition linked to hypoglycemia and/or an overactive thyroid condition.

tikta ghrita — a special Āyurvedic compound of clarified butter with various bitter herbs used for medicinal purposes; bitter ghee

tittiraka — a partridge, used to describe a type of pitta pulse

tribhuja — onyx

tridosha — the three forces within the body; the three bodily humors: air (vāta), fire/ bile (pitta) and water (kapha)

trikatu — an Āyurvedic herbal compound of ginger, black pepper and Piper longum that burns āma, detoxifies the body and improves digestion, absorption and assimilation

U

udāna — pushes upward

udāna vāyu — one of the five subtypes of vāta which moves energy upward and is responsible for exhalation and vomiting. It gives energy, memory and vitality. All upward movement within the body is governed by udāna vāyu.

unmāda — mental disorder; mania or psychosis; psychotic diseases

upa damsha — syphilis

urustambha — paraplegia

ushna — hot; characterized by heat, expansion, cleansing, digestion, anger, hate and judgmentalism

ushtra gati — the camel pulse; indicates aortic stenosis with thickening or narrowing of the aortic valve; felt under the vāta or pitta finger

ūrdhva jatru granthi — hyperthyroidism

V

vāta — one of the three doshas, combining the Space and Air elements; the subtle energy associated with movement. It governs breathing, blinking, muscle and tissue movement, pulsation of the heart, and all movements in the cytoplasm and cell membranes. In balance, *vāta* promotes creativity and flexibility. Out of balance, *vāta* produces fear and anxiety.

vāta gulma — diverticulosis or the formation of empty, balloon-like cul-de-sacs

Vāyavya — a personality type, found at the sixth level of the pulse, indicating someone who is rajasic and emotional with mood swings

vaidūrya — moonstone gemstone

vajra — a variety of diamond found naturally in coal mines that is very difficult to break

vam — the mantra of the second chakra, svādisthāna, located in the pelvic area; the seed sound of the water element

Varuna — a personality type, found at the sixth level of the pulse, indicating someone who is sattvic, loving and compassionate; also, the name of the god of water or the sea

varuna — an opal gemstone, the opal is also called sāgararāja

vega — the rate of the pulse

vepathu — Parkinson's disease or tremors

vijñānam — understanding, comprehension or specialized knowledge

vikruti — the current state of the individual versus the permanent constitution (prakruti); it may also denote disorder

vilambikā nādi — a nādi located at the sciatic nerve

visarpa — erysipelas

vishama agni — an irregular state of agni; the imbalanced fire or metabolism; the gastric fire being sometimes strong, sometimes weak, sometimes fast, sometimes slow, resulting in imbalanced digestion

Vishnu — the Supreme Lord; the All-pervading One without a second; the divine qualities are: knowledge, strength, lordship, power, virility and splendor; the Preserver; the second in the Hindu God trinity

vishva — universe, part of a synonym for the pulse

visphota — herpes zoster or shingles

vishuddha — the fifth chakra, located at the throat

vyāna — circulates or carries rasa and rakta dhātus, plasma, nutrients, oxygen from one part of the body to another

vyāna vāyu — one of the five vāta subtypes; the vital air; the life-breath which governs the circulation of blood in the body; regulates the nervous, muscular and skeletal systems in the body; responsible for the reflex arc, activity and movement of all joints

vyakta, vyakti — that which is visible, manifest, created; the fifth stage of pathogenesis manifesting as general disease

Y

yakrut — the liver

yakrut roga — liver disorders

yam — the mantra of Air; the seed sound of the Air element; a pleasing, circulating sound

Yama — the name of the god of death; a personality type, found at the sixth level of the pulse, indicating someone who is impartial, withdrawn and introspective

yamas — the first yogic discipline; restraints; abstentions; self-control; the practice of self-restraint: non-injury (non-violence), truthfulness, non-stealing (forgiving theft), celibacy, and non-possession; Vāsishtha says, "Look far, not near. Look toward the highest and not toward that which is less than the highest." Another way of addressing the yamas is: non-violence, truth speaking, abstinence from stealing, celibacy and dis-owning of possessions.

yashava — jade; a success-giving gem

yoga — union of the lower self with the higher self; of the inner with the outer, of mortality with immortality, of logic with love, of the definition with the undefined which happens at sahasrāra within the brain

yoga mudrā — in a sitting posture (lotus) with a forward bend, place the face to the floor; enables the union of the lower self with the higher self

yogi — the enlightened one; the blissful one; one who practices yoga

BIBLIOGRAPHY AND SELECTED READINGS

Bhishagratna, Kaviraj Kunjalal, editor-translator. *Sushruta Samhita.* 4th ed., 2 vols., Chowkhamba Sanskrit Series Office: Varanasi, India, 1991.

Frawley, David. *Ayurvedic Healing.* Morson Publishing: Salt Lake City, 1989.

Frawley, David, and Vasant Lad. *The Yoga of Herbs.* Lotus Press: Santa Fe, 1986.

Lad, Vasant. *Ayurveda: The Science of Self-Healing.* Lotus Press: Santa Fe, 1984.

————. *The Textbook of Ayurveda: Fundamental Principles, Vol. 1.* The Ayurvedic Press: Albuquerque, 2002.

Murthy, K. R. Srikantha, translator. *Sharngadhara Samhita: A Treatise on Ayurveda.* Chaukhambha Orientalia: Varanasi, India, 1984.

Morrison, Judith H. *The Book of Ayurveda: A Holistic Approach to Health and Longevity.* New York: Simon & Schuster Inc., 1995, A Fireside Book.

Sharma, Priyavrat V., editor-translator. *Caraka Samhita.* 4 vols. Chowkhamba Sanskrit Series Office: Varanasi, India, 1981-1994.

Sharma, Ram Karan, and Vaidya Bhagwan Dash, editors-translators. *Caraka Samhita.* 3rd ed., 3 vols. Chowkhamba Sanskrit Series Office: Varanasi, India, 1992.

Svoboda, Robert E. *Ayurveda: Life, Health and Longevity.* Penguin: London, 1992; reprint, The Ayurvedic Press: Albuquerque, 2004.

————. *The Hidden Secret of Ayurveda.* Pune, India, 1980; reprint, The Ayurvedic Press: Albuquerque, 1994.

————. *Prakriti: Your Ayurvedic Constitution.* 2nd ed., Lotus Press: Twin Lakes, 1998.

Vagbhata. *Ashtanga Hridayam,* translated by K. R. Srikantha Murthy. 2 vols. Krishnadas Academy: Varanasi, India, 1991-1992.

INDEX

About the Author

Ayurveda finds its home in the hearts of special beings whose dharma it is to preserve and maintain traditions of wisdom for the purpose of healing themselves and the world. Bridging the gap between the changing philosophies, sciences, and religions of the ages, it is passed down in the various cultures through these dedicated individuals. Vasant Lad's heart is one of the homes for that living flame, and his life and teachings are an expression of Ayurveda's true purpose in the world.

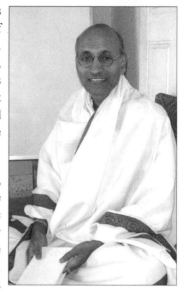

Vasant Lad, BAM&S, MASc, Ayurvedic Physician, brings a wealth of classroom and practical experience to the United States. He received the degree of Bachelor of Ayurvedic Medicine and Surgery (BAM&S) in 1968 from the University of Pune, in Pune, India and a Master of Ayurvedic Science (MASc) in 1980 from Tilak Ayurved Mahavidyalaya in Pune. For 3 years, he served as Medical Director of the Ayurveda Hospital in Pune, India. He also held the position of Professor of Clinical Medicine for seven years at the Pune University College of Ayurvedic Medicine, where he was an instructor for many years. Vasant Lad's academic and practical training includes the study of allopathic medicine (Western Medicine) and surgery as well as traditional Ayurveda. In 1979, he began traveling throughout the United States sharing his knowledge of Ayurveda and, in 1981, he returned to New Mexico to teach Ayurveda. In 1984, he founded and began as Director of The Ayurvedic Institute.

Vasant Lad is the author of 12 books on Ayurveda as well as hundreds of articles and other writings. With over 700,000 copies of his books in print in the US, his work has been translated into more than 20 languages. His books include *Ayurveda, The Science of Self-Healing* and *Secrets of the Pulse* and he is co-author of *The Yoga of Herbs* and *Ayurvedic Cooking for Self-Healing*. His work from Harmony Books, *The Complete Book of Ayurvedic Home Remedies,* is a compendium of classic Ayurvedic treatments for common and chronic ailments. The series of textbooks on Ayurveda. *The Textbook of Ayurveda: Fundamental Principles, Volume 1, The Textbook of Ayurveda: Clinical Assessment, Volume 2,* and *The Textbook of Ayurveda: General Principles of Management and Treatment, Volume 3* cover the topics he teaches in his residential Ayurvedic Studies Programs. He is co-author of a book on marma therapy, *Marma Points of Ayurveda,* and the author of *Applied Marma Therapy Cards,* a flash card study set for marma therapy. Additionally, he teaches the practice of pranayama, breathing exercises, on the DVD *Pranayama for Self-Healing.*

Vasant Lad presently is the Director of The Ayurvedic Institute in Albuquerque, New Mexico and teaches the Ayurvedic Studies Programs, Level 1 and 2, as well as advanced training programs in India each year. Vasant Lad also travels throughout the world, consulting privately and giving seminars on Ayurveda, its history, theory, principles and practical applications..

For more information about Ayurveda, Dr. Lad's books and his school, check our website www.ayurveda.com or contact The Ayurvedic Institute, 11311 Menaul Blvd NE, Albuquerque, NM 87112-0008, (505) 291-9698.